target to table

2nd edition

healthy and delicious meals
one superfood at a time

by kristen brogan and matt johnson

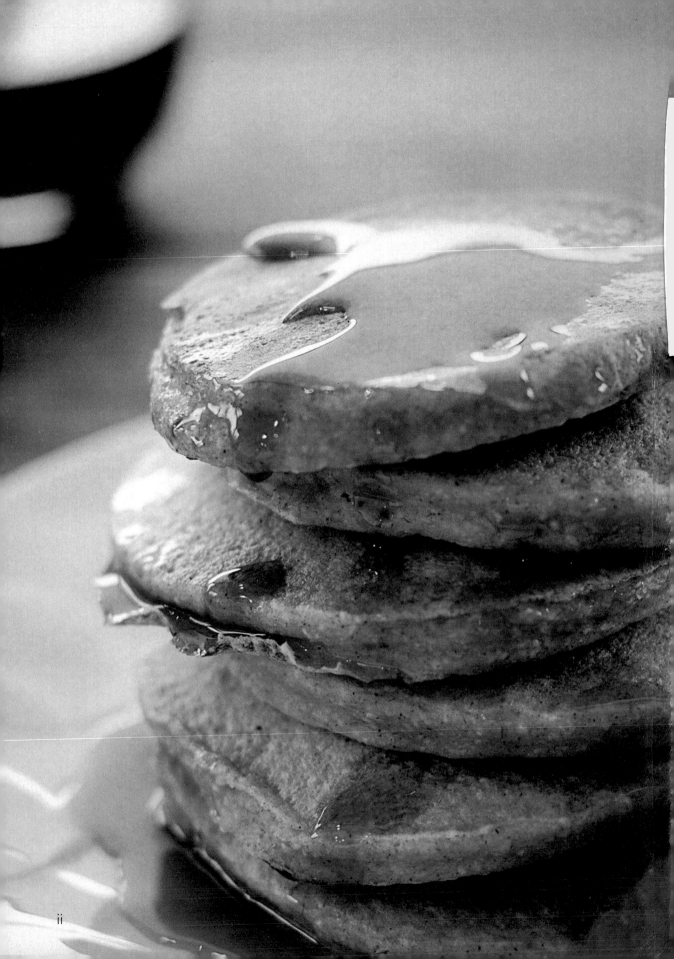

target to table

2nd edition

healthy and delicious meals one superfood at a time

by kristen brogan and matt johnson

Photographs by Matthew Wesener & Ethan Painter
Design by Design 2, Steven Glynn & Lisa Prang

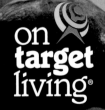

on target living®

ISBN 978-0-9727281-8-8

ontargetliving.com

Photography: Matthew Wesener and Ethan Painter
Design: Design 2, Steven Glynn, and Lisa Prang
Editor: Paula Johnson
Copy editor: Bonney Mayers

We want to thank our amazing mother Paula for teaching us how to make food that combines love and flavor, and especially for all of your editorial, organizational, and technical expertise, and long, hard hours putting this book together…twice. ☺

Thank you to our father Chris for your inspiration, love, and for always encouraging us to find our passion. And for tasting the food. ☺

You both totally rock and we feel so lucky to call you ours.

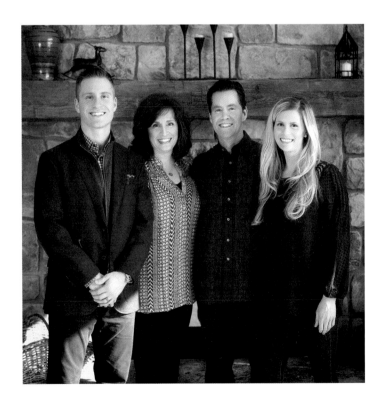

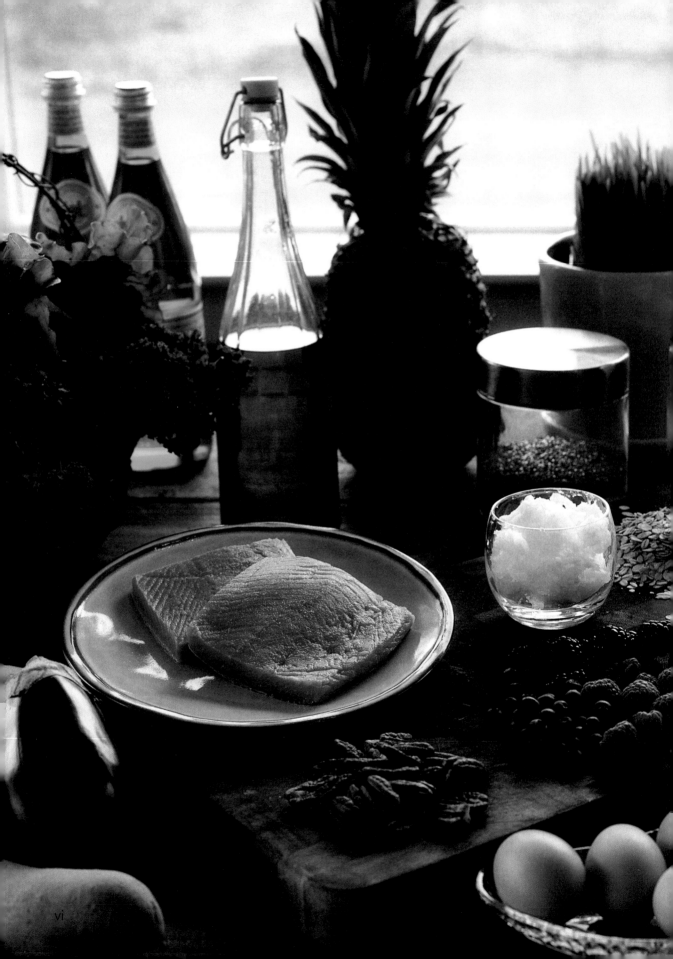

contents

foreword

We at On Target Living are very proud and excited to bring our *Target to Table* cookbook to you! What makes *Target to Table* unique is the quality and taste of each recipe. The recipes are simple, fun to make, extremely healthy, and taste and look fantastic. We wanted to create a cookbook that not only had wonderful recipes to choose from, but also helped educate you the reader along the way—encouraging you to adopt the On Target Living Lifestyle! This is our second cookbook and was conceived around our On Target Living Principles.

The relationship we have with food impacts our lives in so many ways. What we eat, how we eat, when we eat, and why we eat all play a significant role in our health, our energy, our emotions, and our vitality. Food is a big deal to most people!

Many people have beliefs around food that may hinder health, performance, and happiness. Some believe that healthy food tastes bad, carbohydrates make you fat, all calories are created equal, eating healthy costs too much, or healthy cooking requires lots of time. If even one of these statements rings true to you, we hope to dispel those limiting beliefs through recipes that are delicious, satisfying, affordable, and easy to make.

I learned at a young age the power of food and the tremendous impact it can have on your life! I developed major skin problems which started around the age of 8 and continued into my early 20's. I was prescribed oral medications and topical creams, but nothing seemed to work. The doctors told my parents, "Your son just has sensitive skin." I did not have sensitive skin—it was my poor diet wreaking havoc with my skin. As I started learning more about nutrition and improved my diet, my skin problems slowly disappeared.

Do you remember the song in the classic movie *Mary Poppins* that included the words medicine and sugar? Mary Poppins would sing over and over, "Just a spoon full of sugar helps the medicine go down." Hippocrates once said, "Let Food Be Your Medicine and Medicine Be Your Food." Food is a powerful medicine, and when chosen and prepared correctly, there's no need for the sugar!

In 2006, after working in the health and fitness industry for over twenty years and logging more than 20,000 hours of one-on-one coaching, I decided to take my message out on the road and founded On Target Living. I began traveling the country speaking to corporations, associations, and schools, sharing the On Target Living Lifestyle—REST | EAT | MOVE.

I learned a long time ago that the greatest results are found by working toward a balanced lifestyle that includes getting enough rest, fueling your body with high quality foods and beverages, and moving your body on a daily basis. Nothing fancy—just sustainable lifestyle habits that can be enjoyable, repeatable, and most importantly—create amazing results!

The On Target Living brand is based off the Food Target. I developed the Food Target in 1994 to help people learn how to easily upgrade their food choices, focusing on food quality not just calories! The Food Target focuses on a balance of carbohydrates, proteins, and fats while incorporating an assessment of the quality of their nutrients. The lowest nutritional value foods are located on the outside red area of the Food Target. The highest quality foods, foods in their most natural state including many superfoods, are closer to the green center of the Target.

Superfoods are nutritionally dense foods that keep the body healthy and help you perform at your best. Today my nutritional plan includes many superfoods, such as wheatgrass, spirulina/chlorella, cod liver oil, flaxseeds, cacao nibs, coconut, pumpkin seeds, hemp seeds, macadamia nuts, Brazil nuts, almonds, white figs, dried mango, oatmeal, greens, sweet potatoes, broccoli, dark cherries, raspberries, lemons, and limes.

Our mission at On Target Living is to help people live a healthy and happy life by adopting a healthy lifestyle. Our mantra is "Small Steps to Healthy Living!"

Our number one goal in *Target to Table* is to share our passion and love for food with you and others who want to have food that is truly healthy, energizing, simple, easy, fun, and most importantly, tastes fantastic!

I would like to end by thanking my kids Kristen and Matt, my wife Paula, Bonney our editor, Cindy our designer, and Matt our photographer. All did a wonderful job putting this cookbook together. It really was a team effort.

Wishing you a lifetime of Health & Happiness—Bon Appétit!

Chris Johnson
Founder and CEO
On Target Living

introduction

Born one minute apart, we were no ordinary siblings. Our upbringing was no less unusual. Under our father's influence we were weaned on flaxseeds, cod liver oil, and other freakishly healthy foods. Yuck, right? We didn't know any better.

Our mother, however, taught us how to cook. By the time we were eight years old, we were preparing family dinners once a week and "busting suds" on our nights off. Our family bond was forged celebrating tasty creations and fighting over failures.

It was during childhood that our father Chris Johnson created the Food Target that we know and love. Visually, the concept was and remains simple. The closer the ring is to the center, the healthier the foods. At the very center are the healthiest foods - the superfoods. We came to understand the Target was much more than a colorful circle. See Food Target page xii.

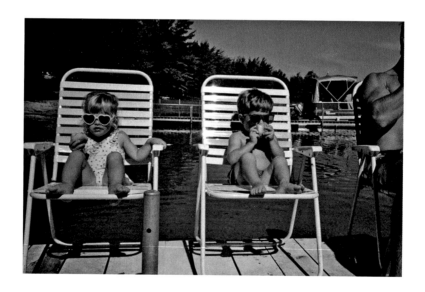

As we grew older, with a refrigerator stocked full of superfoods, we learned how to make food actually taste good and created meals that were healthy and delicious. We started weeding out the less nutritious ingredients from our family's famed recipes and adding *one superfood at a time.*

Why butter? Why not virgin coconut oil?

Why processed sugar? Raw organic honey is plenty sweet.

Why chocolate chips? How about cacao nibs?

The Food Target was working its magic. We were taking "Small Steps to Healthy Living." We like to think that many recipes were improved and others inspired from this undertaking.

In *Target to Table*, we teamed up to share our culinary repertoire with you. Not all of these recipes call for true superfoods, but they will get you started on your quest to move towards the center of the Food Target. Who says healthy cooking can't be fun, delicious and easy all at the same time. Heck, we have a 3-ingredient recipe for banana ice cream!

Creating healthy and delicious meals one superfood at a time means taking those small steps at the store and in the kitchen to develop healthy, lifelong eating habits for you and your family.

From Target to Table, we hope you enjoy these recipes as much as we do!

Kristen Brogan & Matt Johnson

food target

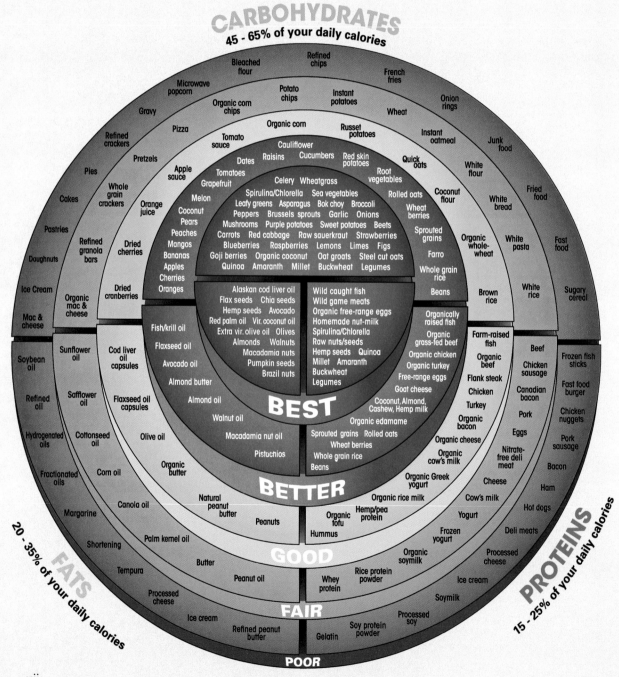

CARBOHYDRATES
45 - 65% of your daily calories

FATS
20 - 35% of your daily calories

PROTEINS
15 - 25% of your daily calories

BEST
BETTER
GOOD
FAIR
POOR

a guide to getting the target to your table

This section includes principles to get you from the shopping cart to the plate. We have provided a basic 101 education on nutrition, digestion, how to read a food label, when to buy organic, what cooking oils to use, and more.

We have chosen not to include the nutritional breakdown for our recipes. That's because the closer you eat to the center of the Food Target the less likely you are to overeat, and therefore you don't have to worry about counting calories, or anything else for that matter. Since the center green circle foods are closer to the "Source", they keep you feeling more nourished and satisfied.

superfoods 101

Superfoods are nutrient-rich foods, such as fruits, vegetables, ancient grains, healthy fats, and lean proteins, considered to be especially beneficial for health and well-being. The focus of this cookbook is to help you learn how to gradually replace not-so-healthy ingredients with more nutritious items such as the superfoods found in the center green circles of the Food Target. See Food Target at left.

the source 101

Source (sôrs, sōrs)
n.
1. The point at which something springs into being or from which it derives or is obtained.
    American Heritage Dictionary

On Target Living bases its teachings on three principles: the Source, Cellular Health, and pH Balance*.

The first of these principles is the Source. Almost every food we eat today is derived from one of the three oldest foods on the planet: grass, algae, and sea vegetables. No one wants to base a diet exclusively on these three foods. However, if you focus on eating foods that are as close to their natural source as possible, you will be practicing the Source principle. So if you are looking for the most nutritious, inexpensive, less processed foods, then the closer you are to the Source the better.

The diagram on page 2 illustrates the progression of food from its original source to a more processed source.

* For more information about On Target Living, visit *ontargetliving.com*.

THE REAL THING ➡		MORE PROCESSED*
APPLE	APPLESAUCE	APPLE JUICE
TOMATO	SALSA	KETCHUP
OAT GROATS	ROLLED OATS	INSTANT OATMEAL
FLAXSEEDS	FLAXSEED OIL	FLAXSEED OIL CAPSULES
SPROUTED BREAD	WHOLE WHEAT BREAD	WHITE BREAD
SWEET POTATOES	WHITE POTATOES	FAST FOOD FRIES
ORGANIC CHICKEN	CHICKEN	CHICKEN NUGGETS
WILD-CAUGHT FISH	FARM-RAISED FISH	FISHSTICKS

When buying more processed foods like breadcrumbs, cereals, chips, crackers, condiments, broths, soups, etc., choose an organic variety if available.

nutrition 101*

Nutrition is the process of absorbing nutrients from food and processing them in the body in order to keep you healthy and nourished. When you eat or drink, the body breaks down the nutrients and uses them for fuel, growth, and repair. Even with all of the food we currently consume in the United States, it still may be possible to be deficient in valuable nutrients.

There are two types of nutritional deficiencies:

• A primary nutrient deficiency occurs when the body lacks a specific nutrient, such as vitamin C, iodine, zinc, magnesium, or omega-3 fats.

• A secondary deficiency occurs when the body fails to absorb or utilize the foods or beverages consumed. Eating closer to the Source will ensure the nutrient absorption of these higher quality foods.

The closer you eat to the Source, the less likely you will be to have a nutrient deficiency.

*See *On Target Living: A Guide to a Life of Balance, Energy, & Vitality* for more information.

digestion 101

Ninety percent of our immune system is based on our digestive health. We have seen an explosion in the amount of digestive health problems, from acid reflux to irritable bowel, constipation, diarrhea, gluten intolerance, food allergies, bloating and gas, skin problems, asthma, cancer, headaches, low energy, inflammation, and type-2 diabetes. The digestive aids aisle in most grocery stores and pharmacies continues to expand.

Having a balanced pH in the digestive tract is crucial for optimal digestion and absorption. The stomach needs to be acidic, the small intestine more alkaline, and the large intestine a neutral pH. Balancing pH may take some time if you are currently consuming too many processed, acidic foods and beverages. If your body is too acidic, you will leach out vital minerals including calcium, magnesium, and iodine. Consuming more alkaline-based foods and beverages is your first step in balancing your pH, along with daily exercise and controlling your stress. See pH table page 5.

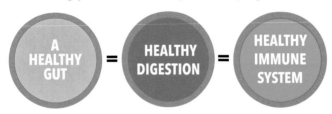

Tips to Improve Digestion and Gut Health

- Avoid processed foods.
- Drink half your body weight in ounces of water every day.
- Chew your food.
- Avoid liquid diets. They do not stimulate the digestive enzymes produced from chewing and can bypass many of the gastrointestinal pathways.
- Eat more "live" foods. An apple turns brown when you bite into it because it is a live food containing enzymes.
- Include fermented foods, such as kefir, kombucha, kimchee, napa cabbage, and sauerkraut.
- Balance your pH by eating more alkaline forming foods such as fruits and vegetables. See pH table page 5.
- Control your stress with exercise, deep breathing, and sleep.
- Eat foods high in chlorophyll, such as wheatgrass, spirulina/chlorella, and leafy greens.
- Add some "friendly bacteria" to the gut by taking a daily probiotic.
- Get sunlight.
- Get up and move.

Gut Superfoods

- Ginger
- Turmeric
- Mint leaves
- Licorice root
- Organic coconut
- Organic virgin coconut oil
- Spirulina/Chlorella
- Wheatgrass juice
- Raw apple cider vinegar

Gut Villains

- Non-organic meat and dairy products
- HFCS (high fructose corn syrup)
- GMOs (genetically modified organisms)
- MSG (monosodium glutamate)
- Synthetic colors
- Artificial or "natural" flavors and sweeteners
- Gluten
- Antibiotics
- Medications
- DPA (diphenylamine) – the wax coating on apples
- Chlorine found in tap water
- Potassium bromate in bread
- Stress
- Lack of exercise
- Lack of sleep

To maintain a balanced pH, shoot for 65 to 70 percent of all your food and beverage sources coming from the alkaline portion of the pH table.

pH table

		More alkaline	Least alkaline	Least acidic	More acidic	Most acidic
Condiments Spices Sweeteners	baking soda, sea salt	cinnamon, most spices, molasses	most herbs, rice syrup	curry, honey, maple syrup, stevia/ agave nectar	vanilla, MSG, Splenda, organic sugar	nutmeg, table salt, pudding, jam/jelly, artificial sweeteners, sugar, cocoa
Beverages	mineral water, lemon/lime water	spring/artesian water, green tea	tap water, ginger tea, herbal tea	purified water, white tea, organic coffee, red wine	distilled water, black tea, white wine	soda pop, energy drinks, coffee, alcohol/beer
Dairy Plant-Based Milk		human breast, almond, & hazelnut milks	ghee, rice, oat, hemp, & coconut milks	butter, yogurt, goat milk, goat cheese	casein, organic cow's milk, soy milk, cottage cheese	ice cream, cow's milk, processed cheese
Meat Seafood Eggs			fish	shrimp, turkey/chicken, game meat, eggs	pork, veal, lean red meat	lobster, hot dogs, deli meat, fast-food, burgers
Grains Cereal			wild rice, quinoa, oats, farro	brown rice, amaranth, millet, kashi	wheat, white rice, rye, spelt	barley, corn
Nuts Oils	pumpkin seeds	almonds, cod liver oil, evening primrose oil, sesame seeds	flaxseed oil, extra virgin olive oil, organic virgin coconut oil, most seeds	pine nuts, safflower oil, almond	sesame oil, peanuts	pecans, brazil nuts, palm kernel oil, fried food, lard, walnuts
Beans Legumes	lentils			pinto beans, lima beans, kidney beans	navy/red beans, split peas, white beans, beans, most legumes	soybeans, tempeh, chickpeas
Vegetables	sea vegetables, broccoli, yams, barley grass, wheatgrass, asparagus, sweet potato, kale, parsley	eggplant, bell peppers, cauliflower, collard greens, garlic sprouts, cabbage, pumpkin	squash, lettuce, beets, cucumber, brussels sprouts	spinach, zucchini, string beans	peas, carrots	
Fruits	lime, pineapple, nectarine, watermelon, raspberries, tangerine	apple, kiwi, peach, blackberries, grapefruit, melon, mango, lemon, avocado	orange, banana, blueberries, strawberries	dried fruit, figs, dates, plum, coconut		

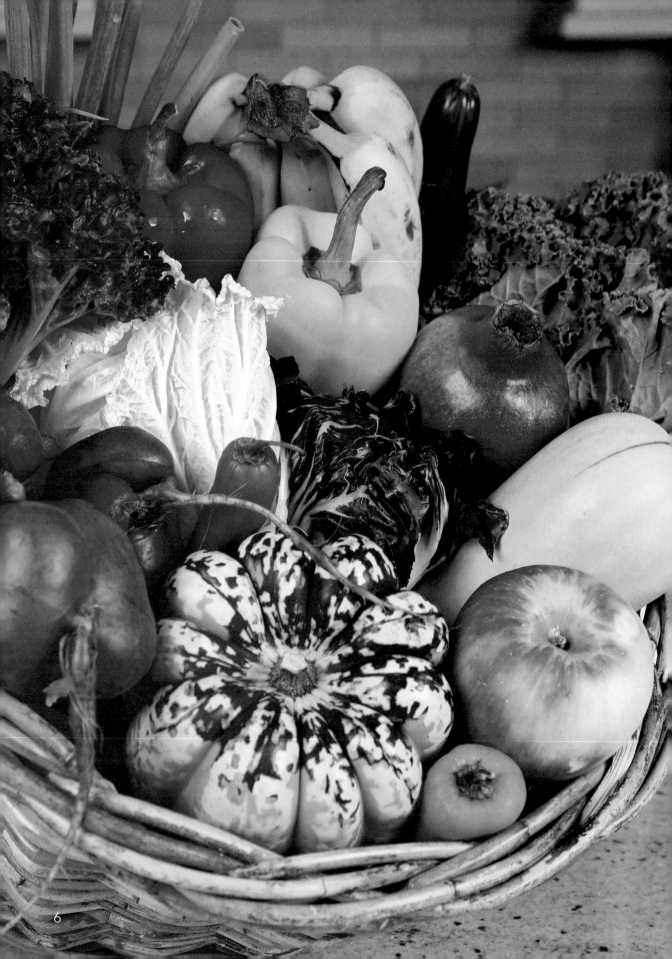

gluten-free 101

Gluten is the protein found in grains such as wheat, rye, and barley. Gluten is found in products such as breads, pizza, pasta, baked goods, cereals, and many processed foods, salad dressings, and sauces. The protein in gluten may be difficult for the body to break down if a person has digestion issues leading to gluten intolerance. Many people are truly gluten intolerant. However, the reason most people have problems breaking down gluten may be due to weak digestion.

Additionally, when you are eating foods closer to the center of the Food Target and the Source, you tend to naturally eat gluten-free. Here's a look at some foods that are naturally gluten-free.

Fruits	Buckwheat	Seeds
Vegetables	Wheatgrass	flaxseeds, chia seeds,
Quinoa	Corn	hemp seeds
Oats	Potatoes	Healthy fats
Millet	Beans	coconut, olive & fish oil
Teff	Nuts	Meat
Rice		Seafood

Question:
   If you remove gluten from a product, is that closer or further from the source?
Answer:
   Further...makes you wonder: is gluten really the problem?

grains 101

Grain-free may be the new craze, but for most people a grain-free diet offers few benefits. In fact, it may even bring unwanted results, such as a deficiency in B vitamins, essential minerals, and problems with brain function and sleep. This way of eating is also difficult to maintain long term.

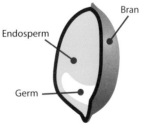

ANATOMY OF A GRAIN

The complex of B vitamins includes eight different vitamins. Whole grains serve as a good source of several B vitamins, including thiamin, riboflavin, niacin, and folate. Thiamin, riboflavin and niacin help your body efficiently break down carbohydrates to use for energy. Folic acid, also known as folate or vitamin B-9, supports the formation and maintenance of new cells. Getting the recommended 400 mcg of folic acid per day, according to the Institute of Medicine's Food and Nutrition Board, is especially important for women of childbearing age, as a deficiency may cause birth defects during the early weeks of pregnancy.

Whole grains also contain essential vitamins such as potassium, magnesium, zinc, and iron. Potassium supports normal heart function, helping to control blood pressure. Magnesium helps to absorb calcium and relax the mind and body helping to improve sleep. Zinc is important for cell metabolism and hormonal balance, while iron is needed to produce proteins and enzymes necessary for the body.

In general, grains serve as a good source of carbohydrates, the type of macronutrient the body uses for energy and brain food. Your body needs at least 400 calories a day from grains for optimal brain function. Because the outermost portion of the grain contains the majority of the vitamins, minerals, and fiber, eating whole grains that contain the bran, germ, and endosperm intact is healthier than eating refined grains that have had the bran and germ removed.

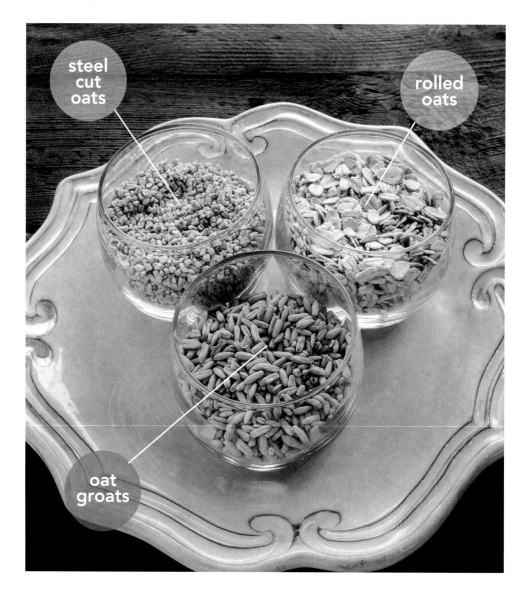

steel cut oats

rolled oats

oat groats

taste 101

Taste continues to be first and foremost when it comes to the way people think about food. Not far behind is nutrition and health. Most people want to eat food that is healthy, but they are not willing to sacrifice taste. As you will see from this cookbook, healthy food can taste great!

There are five types of receptors on the tongue that sense the flavors we taste: sour, sweet, salty, bitter, and umami. Each of these flavors can act on its own, but how they interact with each other is essential to making food taste delicious. Activation of any one taste will enhance another taste. Blending these tastes together is the foundation for great tasting healthy recipes.

All of these tastes can be found in the following fruits and vegetables.

Taste	Foods
Sour	Citrus fruits (lemons, limes, oranges), kiwi, blueberries
Sweet	Apples, watermelon, grapes, pears, carrots, sweet potatoes, beets
Salty	Celery, rhubarb, bok choy, sea vegetables
Bitter	Leafy greens (arugula, kale)
Umami*	Tomatoes, mushrooms, raw corn, truffle oil

Umami is a Japanese word that describes a meaty or savory taste. Tomatoes and mushrooms are high in free-form glutamate which provides a natural umami flavor. Roasting or sautéing will further intensify this flavor.

All tastes contribute to a well-balanced diet as the foods that make up each contain several essential nutrients. Usually when all five tastes are incorporated into a meal, you feel satisfied and less likely to overeat. Adding a squeeze of lemon to cooked dishes can quickly satisfy the sour taste, while adding a side of greens will fulfill the bitter taste.

organic 101

Organic food is produced without using pesticides, herbicides, fungicides, antibiotics, and fertilizers made from synthetic ingredients. Organic meat, poultry, eggs, and dairy products come from animals that are not fed or given pesticides, growth hormones, or antibiotics.

Try to buy these products whenever possible to avoid consuming residual pesticides, antibiotics, and growth hormones.

- Organic dairy (milk, cottage cheese, cheese, yogurt)
- Organic poultry
- Wild game
- Grass-fed beef
- Wild-caught fish

When choosing to buy organic fruits and vegetables, start with the "Dirty Dozen." These are fruits and vegetables that have the highest pesticide levels. These become more important if you plan to eat the skin on these products.

Dirty Dozen (high pesticide levels)

- Apples
- Bell peppers
- Carrots
- Celery
- Cherries
- Grapes
- Lettuce
- Nectarines
- Peaches
- Pears
- Spinach
- Strawberries

Cleaner Dozen (low pesticide levels)

- Asparagus
- Avocado
- Bananas
- Broccoli
- Cauliflower
- Kiwi
- Mangos
- Onions
- Peas
- Pineapple
- Sweet potatoes
- Tomatoes

Say "No" to GMO

GMOs (genetically modified organisms) are plants or animals created through gene-splicing techniques. This technology combines DNA from different species, creating combinations of plant and animal genes that cannot be found in nature or in traditional crossbreeding. GMOs were developed to offer benefits to the consumer such as increased yield, greater protection from herbicides and drought, and enhanced nutrition. A growing body of evidence shows that the claims of many of these consumer benefits are not true, and GMOs have been connected with health problems, environmental damage, and violation, of farmers and consumers' rights.

Current GMO High-Risk Foods

- Alfalfa
- Canola
- Corn
- Soy
- Sugar beets

Common Ingredients Derived from GMO High-Risk Crops

- Amino acids, aspartame, ascorbic acid, vitamin C, citric acid
- Sodium citrate, ethanol, flavorings, high fructose corn syrup
- Hydrolyzed vegetable protein, lactic acid, maltodextrins, MSG
- Sucrose, textured vegetable protein, xanthan gum, vitamins, and yeast products

These GMO ingredients are in everything from bread, salad dressings, crackers, frozen pizza, soda pop—almost everywhere you look.

To avoid consuming GMO products, eat more organic whole foods, fewer processed foods, beverages, and supplements, and look for the non-GMO Verified Seal. That seal features brands enrolled in the Non-GMO Project, a nonprofit organization committed to providing consumers with clearly labeled Non-GMO food choices.

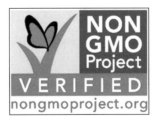

Notice the PLU label on the fruits and vegetables

- If it has a **5-digit code** and begins with a **9**, it means that it was organically grown.
- If the label has a **4-digit code**, it means that it was conventionally grown but not organic.
- If it has a **5-digit code** and begins with an **8**, it means that it was genetically modified. However, producers are not yet required to label GMO foods so foods with a 4-digit PLU code could contain GMOs.

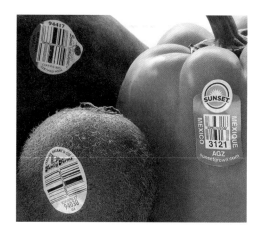

cooking 101

Here are some tips to use while cooking and eating your way through the book.

- Use the Food Target as a guide for shopping and cooking. The center green circles contain the most nutritious and most flavorful foods.
- Choose extra virgin or expeller pressed oils such as extra virgin olive oil or virgin coconut oil. See Cooking Oil Guide at right.
- When using salt, choose natural sea salt. Celtic sea salt contains the most iodine.
- Use one-ingredient foods as much as possible, as they provide the most flavor and nutrition. For example: oats, quinoa, broccoli, apples
- If choosing packaged foods, avoid products that have a long ingredient list or unfamiliar ingredients.
- Choose "natural" products that are minimally processed:

  No high fructose corn syrup, refined sugars, or artificial sweeteners

  No hydrogenated oils (trans fats)

  No refined flours or milled grains

  No artificial food colorings, flavorings, or preservatives

  No GMOs

Cooking Oil Guide

This cooking oil chart includes the highest quality oils best used in cooking. Higher quality oil equals more nutrition and flavor.

For high temperature cooking, select cooking oil with a high smoke point. Heating an oil above its smoke point produces toxic fumes and harmful free radicals. Usually the more refined the oil the higher the smoke point. High quality oils tend to have lower smoke points and contain more flavor and nutrition.

Oil	Smoke Point	Uses
Pumpkin Seed Oil	320°F	Best used for no heat cooking; dressings, dips
Walnut Oil (Unrefined)	320°F	Salad dressings Add to cold dishes to enhance flavor
Organic Virgin Coconut Oil	350°F	Low to medium heat cooking, sautéing, salad oils/dressings Substitute for processed oils/butters
Red Palm Oil (Virgin, Unrefined)	350°F	Medium heat cooking, sautéing and frying, cooking/drizzling on popcorn
Extra Virgin Olive Oil	375°F	Low to medium heat cooking, sautéing, salad oils/dressings Substitute for processed vegetable oils
Macadamia Nut Oil	390°F	Low heat cooking, sautéing, salad dressings
Almond Oil	420°F	Medium-high heat cooking, sautéing, frying
Grapeseed Oil	420°F	Medium-high heat cooking, sautéing, grilling Mild flavor
Sesame Oil	450°F	High heat cooking, deep frying
Avocado Oil	520°F	High heat cooking, sautéing, frying

healthy food substitutions 101

Ingredient	Healthy Substitution
Bacon	Organic bacon, turkey bacon
Bouillon cubes	Chicken broth, vegetable broth, bone broth
Bottled dressings	Extra virgin olive oil mixed with balsamic vinegar or lemon juice
Bread/wraps for sandwiches	Lettuce wraps, collard greens , coconut wraps, sprouted grain wraps
Breadcrumbs	Shredded coconut, coconut flour, quinoa flour, almond meal, hemp seeds
Butter/oil in baking	Organic butter from grass-fed cows, organic virgin coconut oil, puréed pumpkin, mashed bananas, applesauce
Butter/oil in cooking	Organic butter from grass-fed cows, organic virgin coconut oil
Buttermilk (1 cup)	1 tablespoon lemon juice plus enough organic almond milk to make 1 cup. Let sit 5 minutes.
Canned fruit in heavy syrup	Fresh fruit or canned fruit in 100% fruit juice
Cheese	Organic cheese, goat cheese, sheep feta
Chips	Kale chips
Chocolate chips	Dark chocolate chips, cacao nibs
Coffee	Teeccino herbal coffee, organic coffee, organic green tea, herbal teas
Cornstarch/thickeners	Chia seeds, sea vegetable flakes (agar agar), potato starch
Crackers & cheese	Veggies & hummus
Cream/creamers	Organic dairy creamers, cashew milk, almond milk, coconut milk
Egg	1 tablespoon ground flaxseeds mixed with 3 tablespoons water or 1 tablespoon chia seeds with 6 tablespoons water Let sit 10 minutes. ¼ cup puréed prunes, pumpkin, squash, or applesauce
Frosting	Organic powdered sugar, Coconut Butter Frosting (see recipe page 187)

Ingredient	Healthy Substitution
Ice cream	Banana ice cream (see recipe page 188.)
Jam/Jelly	Organic pure fruit spreads; apple, cherry or grape butter
Mashed white potatoes	Mashed sweet potatoes, cauliflower, or root vegetables
Mayonnaise	Mashed avocado or organic nonfat Greek yogurt mixed with 1 teaspoon organic sugar, 1 teaspoon apple cider vinegar, salt & black pepper
Microwave popcorn	Popcorn prepared in virgin coconut oil (see recipe page 51)
Milk	Almond milk, cashew milk, -coconut milk, oat milk, hemp milk
Peanut butter	Natural peanut butter, cashew butter, almond butter
Pectin (in jam)	Chia gel (chia seeds mixed with water in a 1:6 ratio)
Salt	Herbs & spices, garlic & onion powder, ground dried mushrooms, kelp, Celtic sea salt
Sour cream	Organic nonfat plain Greek yogurt
Soy Sauce	Bragg's Liquid Aminos, coconut aminos
Sugar	Homemade applesauce (see recipe page 54.), puréed dried fruit like dates and figs, honey, agave nectar, maple syrup, molasses, stevia, vanilla extract
Sugary beverages/cocktails	Water with fresh fruit, such as sliced lemons, limes or oranges. (see mineral water cocktail recipe page 20.)
Traditional pie crust	Raw fruit and nut crust (see recipe page 192), Oatmeal Crust (see recipe page 44)
White bread	Whole wheat, whole grain, sprouted bread/wraps
White flour	White whole wheat flour, almond flour, coconut flour
White pasta	Whole grain pasta, spaghetti squash, black bean pasta, lentil pasta, mung bean pasta, spiral cut zucchini
White rice	Wild or long-grain rice, quinoa

smoothie 101

Use this as a guide to build your perfect smoothie. Simply start with a liquid, toss in fruit, throw in greens, build in protein, and add healthy fats. Bump up the nutrition even more by adding "Superpower Smoothie Superfoods" from the list at right.

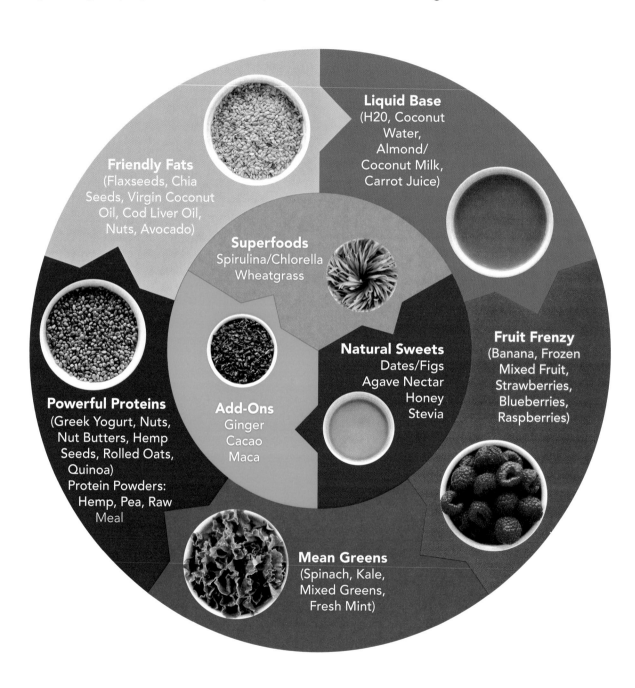

Liquid Base
(H20, Coconut Water, Almond/ Coconut Milk, Carrot Juice)

Friendly Fats
(Flaxseeds, Chia Seeds, Virgin Coconut Oil, Cod Liver Oil, Nuts, Avocado)

Superfoods
Spirulina/Chlorella Wheatgrass

Fruit Frenzy
(Banana, Frozen Mixed Fruit, Strawberries, Blueberries, Raspberries)

Natural Sweets
Dates/Figs Agave Nectar Honey Stevia

Powerful Proteins
(Greek Yogurt, Nuts, Nut Butters, Hemp Seeds, Rolled Oats, Quinoa)
Protein Powders: Hemp, Pea, Raw Meal

Add-Ons
Ginger Cacao Maca

Mean Greens
(Spinach, Kale, Mixed Greens, Fresh Mint)

Superpower Smoothie Superfoods

Cacao

Cacao is the raw unprocessed form of chocolate and is high in magnesium, manganese, zinc, and iron. Cacao has many benefits including brain health, mood enhancement, heart health, weight loss, and improved energy. It can also enhance relaxation and promote a better night's sleep. Because it is high in magnesium, it has also been shown to build muscle and aid in muscle recovery. Did you know that cacao also contains more antioxidants than red wine, green tea, and blueberries?

Figs

This dried fruit is high in the calming mineral magnesium, which helps relax the mind and body. Figs are also high in fiber, helping to promote a healthy digestion.

Almonds

This popular nut is high in calcium needed to build strong bones, improve muscle function, and absorb magnesium.

Brazil Nuts

These nuts are high in selenium, a trace mineral essential to immune and thyroid function. Brazil nuts are also high in magnesium which helps with the functioning of muscles, production of protein, and absorption of energy from food.

Superseeds (Flax, Chia, Hemp)

Flaxseeds and chia seeds are high in omega 3s (ALA), which provide antiviral, antifungal, antibacterial, and anticancer properties. Hemp seeds are also high in omega 3s (LA and GLA), along with being high in protein.

Coconut

Coconuts are a healthy saturated fat high in lauric, capric, and caprylic acids, which all have antiviral and antifungal properties contributing to a healthy digestion. Coconuts also contain medium chain fatty acids that can aid in a healthy metabolism.

Leafy Greens

We all know that eating leafy greens provides many benefits, but did you know they are a good source of calcium? Leafy greens are also high in vitamin C, helping to keep your immune system healthy and prevent you from getting sick.

Cod Liver Oil

This omega 3 fat contains EPA and DHA all of which contribute to a healthy heart, brain, hormonal balance, and decreased inflammation. Cod liver oil is also high in vitamin D which is needed to absorb calcium.

Spirulina & Chlorella

This fresh water algae helps to build the immune system, detoxify the body, and improve digestion. Spirulina and chlorella are also high in protein, making it a great source for vegans or protein needs in general.

Maca Powder

This plant powder can boost energy levels and even enhance athletic performance. Maca has also been shown to decrease levels of stress-inducing hormones, cortisol, and adrenaline.

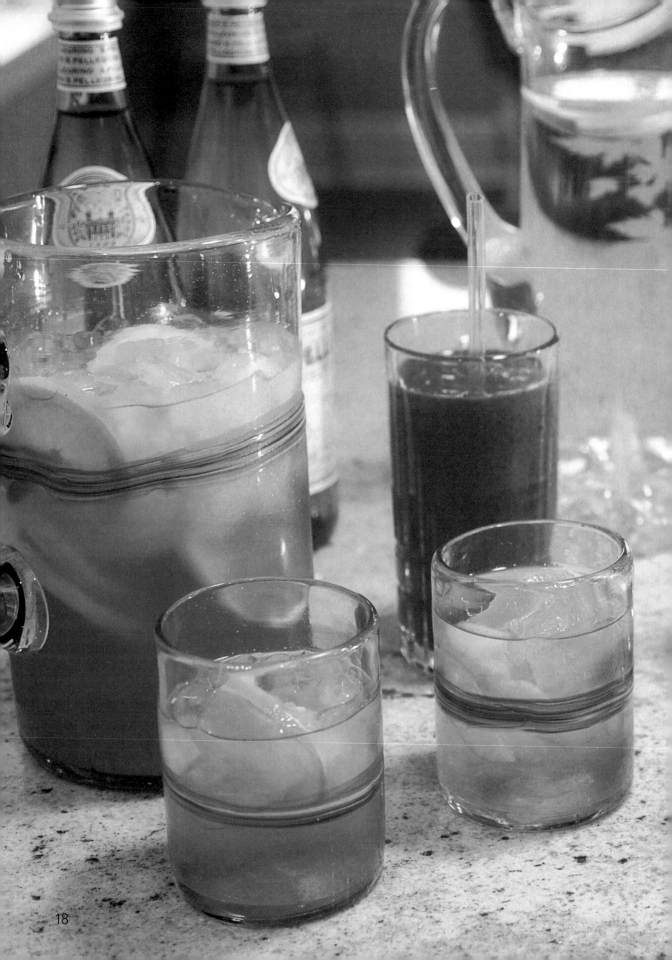

beverages

very berry mineral water cocktail

Serves 4

1 bottle (33.8 ounces) natural sparkling mineral water

8 ounces sparkling juice

1 orange, sliced

1 lemon, sliced

Ice

Combine ingredients in a large pitcher and serve.

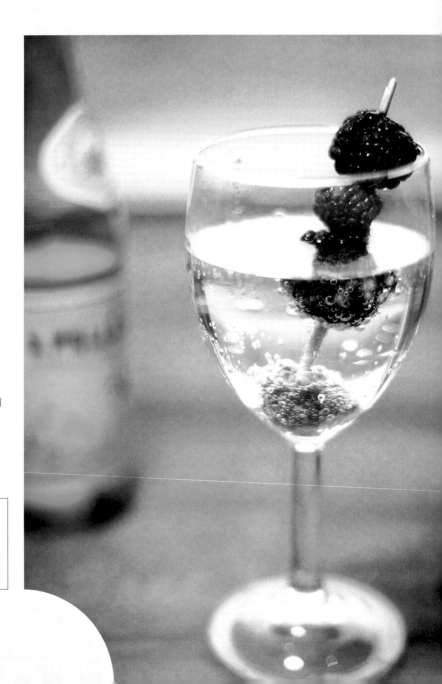

tip ▶ Skewer raspberries, blueberries, and blackberries on a cocktail straw or toothpick, and place in the freezer overnight. Place frozen fruit skewer in your favorite wine or cocktail glass and add carbonated mineral water.

 Mineral Water Cocktail is full of electrolytes, making it a great sports recovery drink to refuel and replenish the body.

detox juice

Serves 2

Combine all ingredients in a juicer and drink immediately.

1 beet, peeled

2 stalks celery

4 carrots

1 apple, cored

1-inch piece fresh ginger, peeled

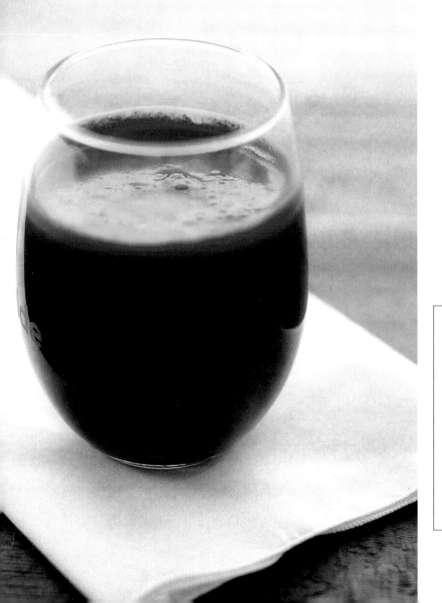

 If you are interested in doing a liquid cleanse/detox, try a broth cleanse instead. Simply make your own by boiling chicken/beef bones or buy organic bone broth; heat, and serve with a side of greens. Bone broths contain more vitamins, minerals, and protein compared to traditional broths/stocks.

8 ounces coconut water

Large handful kale

1 frozen banana

2 dates, pitted

2 tablespoons hempseeds

1 tablespoon ground
flaxseeds

1 tablespoon fresh ginger,
minced (optional)

2 cups almond milk

2 large frozen ripe bananas

1 tablespoon chia seeds

3 tablespoons natural peanut
butter

¼ teaspoon vanilla extract

Ice, if desired

tip▶ Hemp seeds are a great
alternative to protein
powder in your smoothies.

the perfect green smoothie

Serves 1
Mix all ingredients in a blender until smooth.

peanut butter bomb smoothie

Serves 2-3

Mix all ingredients in a blender until smooth.

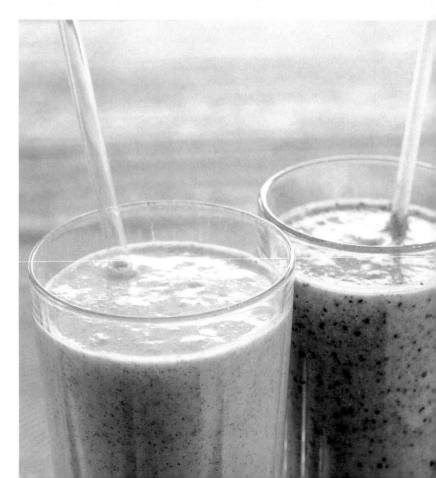

mint chocolate chip smoothie

Serves 2

Add all ingredients to a blender except cacao nibs and blend until smooth. Add in cacao and blend to mix, about 5 seconds. Thin with water if needed. If using frozen bananas, leave out ice.

 This smoothie is loaded in calming magnesium-rich superfoods for better sleep and testosterone boosting superseeds for increasing metabolism and improving performance.

2 bananas

2 cups pure coconut water

¼ cup pumpkin seeds

½ cup unsweetened shredded coconut

¼ cup hemp seeds

4 dates, pitted

1 cup fresh mint leaves

1 cup spinach

1 handful ice

¼ cup cacao nibs

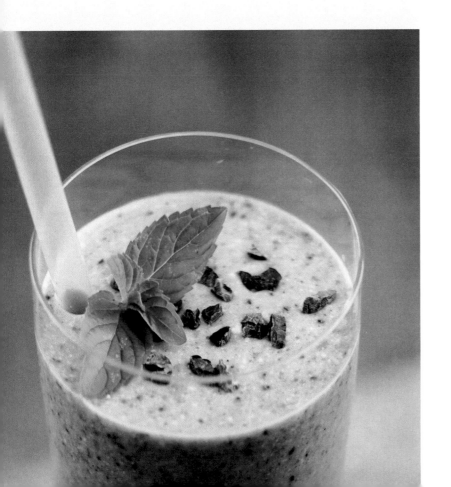

rise & shine smoothie

Serves 3

2 cups water or carrot juice

1 cup kale or spinach

1 banana

2 cups frozen or fresh berries

2 tablespoons chia seeds or ground flaxseeds

2 tablespoons hemp seeds

Mix all ingredients in a blender until smooth.

 Throw flaxseeds or chia seeds into your smoothies for an easy way to add healthy omega 3s to your diet. These super seeds are also high in fiber and protein, and have antiviral properties all contributing to a healthy immune system.

r & r smoothie

Serves 2

1 10-12 ounce bag frozen mixed fruit

1 banana

1 tablespoon cacao nibs

2 cups coconut water

2 dates, pitted (or figs)

2 tablespoons Brazil nuts

2 cups spinach

Combine all ingredients in a blender until smooth.

 Cacao, dates, Brazil nuts, and leafy greens are all high in the calming mineral magnesium, making this a perfect drink for rest and recovery.

homemade coconut milk

Serves 4

Add coconut and water to a blender. Mix on high for 1-2 minutes or until water turns milky. Store in the refrigerator and use within 4 to 5 days. Shake well before using.

1 cup shredded coconut

5-6 cups water

1 teaspoon vanilla extract

 Most store-bought, plant-based milks contain carrageenan, xanthan gum, and other processed stabilizers. You can avoid these types of additives by making your own coconut milk.

molasses & fig almond milk

Serves 5

Place almonds in a glass bowl and cover with water. Soak for 8 hours or overnight. Drain and rinse almonds.

Add almonds, molasses, figs, water, and vanilla extract to blender and mix until smooth.

1 cup raw almonds

1 tablespoon blackstrap molasses

4 dried figs

4 cups water

1 teaspoon vanilla extract (optional)

 Blackstrap molasses and almonds are naturally high in calcium making this a calcium-rich, plant-based milk. One serving provides about 8 grams of protein.

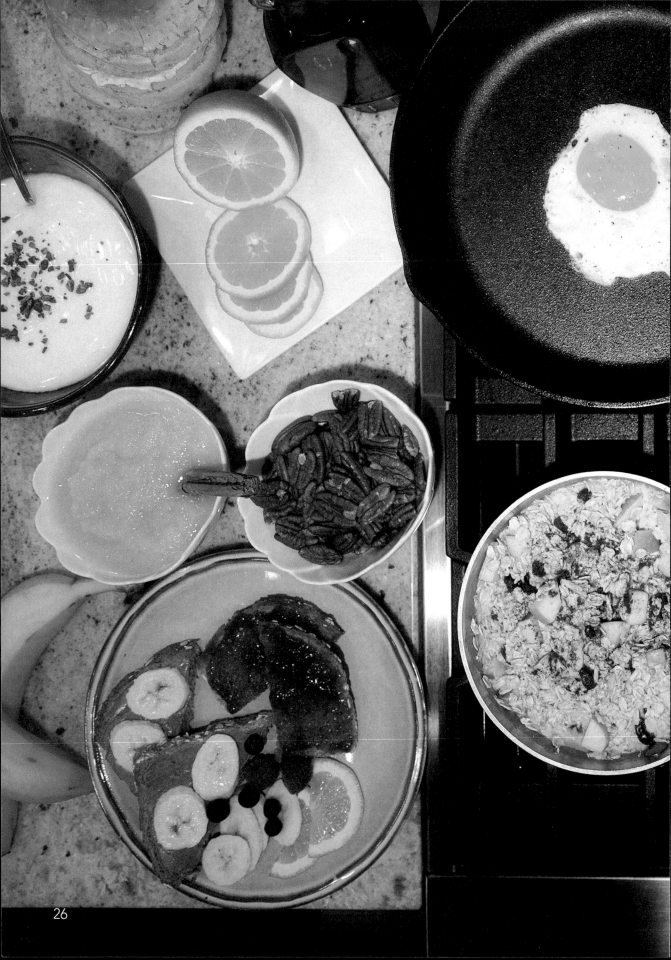

breakfasts

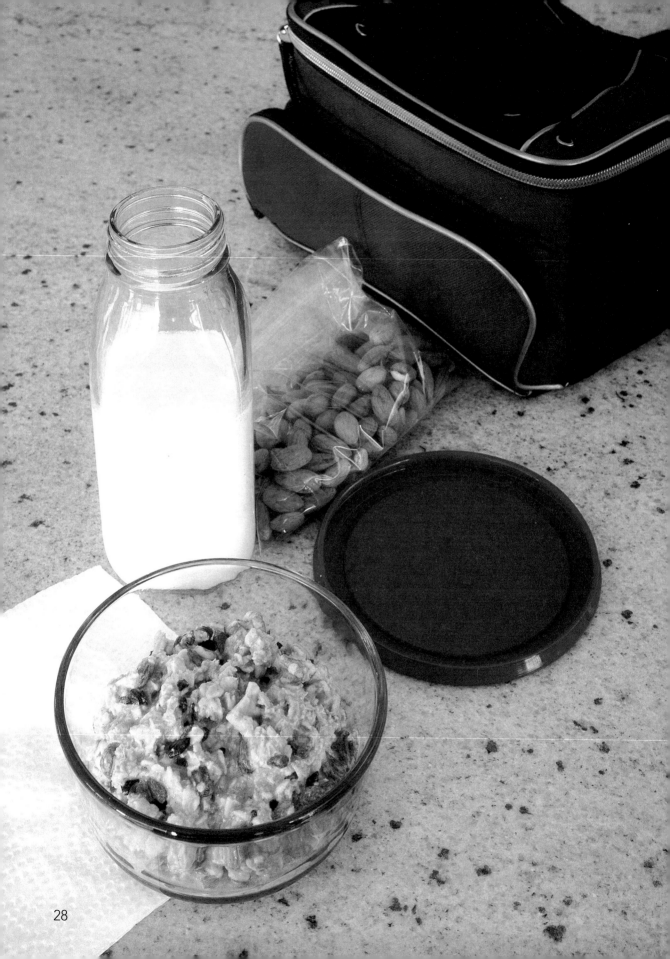

oatmeal on the run

Serves 1

Combine dry ingredients in a small travel container and mix to incorporate. Pour nut milk over oat mixture just to cover. Let soak overnight in the refrigerator. Grab and go in the morning.

½ cup rolled oats

1 teaspoon ground cinnamon

2 tablespoons raisins

2 tablespoons walnuts (can use any nuts)

⅔ cup almond, coconut, or hemp milk (just enough to cover the oat mixture)

chris: *My grandmother turned me on to oatmeal when I was 8 years old. She ate it every morning and lived to age 98. I came up with this recipe for those days when I didn't have time to cook oatmeal in the morning. Now it's my favorite way to eat oatmeal.*

tip▶ You can make a big batch to keep in the refrigerator for the week. Play with the combination of fruit and nuts to your liking.

overnight oats with figs & apples

Serves 4

Rinse oats and soak in cold water for 1 hour.

Drain oats and add to small (1.5 quart) slow cooker. Mix in cinnamon and then stir in 4 cups of water, chopped apples or pears, and figs.

Cook in slow cooker for 7-8 hours or overnight. Serve warm with almond milk.

1 cup oat groats (see page 8 for photo of oat varieties)

1 teaspoon ground cinnamon

4 cups water

1 apple or pear, peeled and chopped

4 dried figs, chopped

tip▶ Oat groats are great but who has the time to cook them? Simply throw them in a slow cooker overnight and breakfast is served! The delicious smell will have you out of bed in seconds and this warm bowl of deliciousness will stick with you until lunch.

superhero breakfast

Serves 8

2 cups traditional quinoa, rinsed and drained

½ cup natural crunchy peanut butter

2 tablespoons honey

1 tablespoon cinnamon

½ cup raisins

Bring quinoa and 4 cups water to a boil.

Lower heat to simmer and cook for 10-15 minutes or until quinoa is al dente, and all the water is absorbed.

While hot, mix in peanut butter, honey, and cinnamon. Stir in raisins.

Serve warm or chilled. Lasts up to 5 days in the refrigerator.

kristen: *I call this a superhero breakfast because it is super healthy and kid-approved!*

 Super-nutrition for a super-hero! Quinoa is an ancient grain high in protein, fiber, and energizing carbohydrates.

teff porridge

Serves 2-3

1 cup teff

4 cups water

1 tablespoon cacao powder (optional)

1 tablespoon honey

Bring water to a boil then add teff and cacao if using.

Boil for 10 minutes then turn to low and simmer for about 15 minutes, stirring frequently.

Drizzle with honey if desired.

 Teff is an ancient grain loaded in protein, iron, calcium, and energizing B vitamins. It is also Gluten-free and easy to digest.

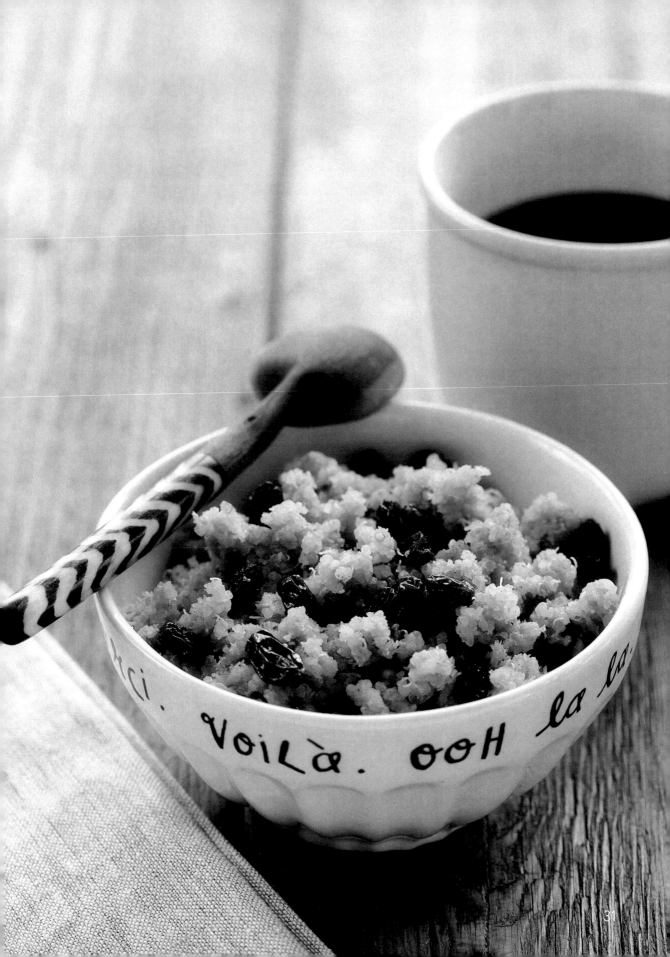

traverse city cherry granola

Serves 8-10

3 cups rolled oats

1 cup unsweetened dried coconut flakes

1 cup pecans, roughly chopped

½ cup dried tart cherries

⅛ cup flaxseeds

Dash of sea salt

Dash of nutmeg

½ cup pure maple syrup

¼ cup virgin coconut oil

1 tablespoon honey

1 teaspoon vanilla extract

Preheat oven to 300°F.

Combine the dry ingredients and mix together (oats, coconut flakes, pecans, cherries, flaxseeds, sea salt, and nutmeg).

In a small saucepan, combine the wet ingredients (syrup, virgin coconut oil, honey, and vanilla extract) until melted. Once melted and mixed, pour over the dry ingredients and mix well.

Grease a large cookie sheet with virgin coconut oil. Spread out mixture onto the cookie sheet.

Bake for 15 minutes. Stir mixture on the cookie sheet and bake for another 15 minutes. While still warm, transfer into a large glass container.

Traverse City, Michigan is known as the cherry capital of the world. With more than 3.8 million tart cherry trees, the Traverse City area produces 70-75% of the tart cherries grown in the United States.

holly: *This is a recipe that I perfected using the Target to Table philosophy. I was not always a "Target to Table" girl, but soon after meeting Matt I started challenging myself to make substitutions based on these principles. Now it's second nature for me to adapt all of my recipes.*

tip ▶ Virgin coconut oil is a great substitute for butter or vegetable oil, providing a nutty coconut flavor when added to dishes. This provides a healthy oil + a healthy sweet.

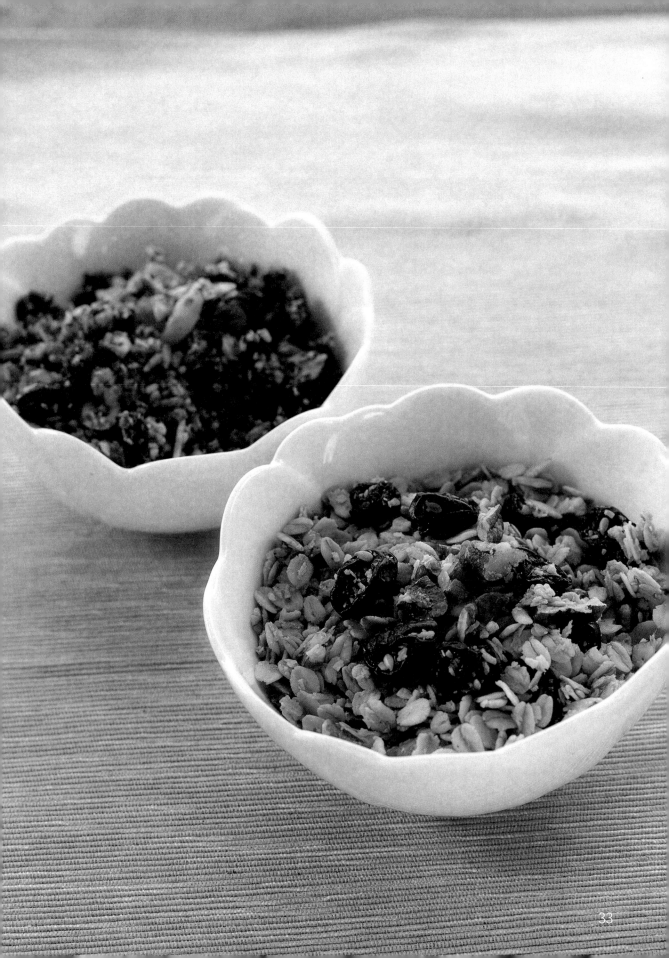

¼ cup chopped pecans

¼ cup sliced almonds or raw almonds

¼ cup sunflower seeds

1 cup steel cut oats

1 tablespoon ground cinnamon

¼ cup virgin coconut oil, melted

¼ cup pure maple syrup

1 tablespoon vanilla extract

¼ cup chia seeds

¼ cup raisins

¼ cup golden raisins

½ cup toasted coconut flakes

nutty seedy granola

Serves 8-10

Spread pecans, almonds, sunflower seeds, and oats evenly on a baking sheet. Bake for 5 minutes.

Remove tray from oven and place nut and oat mixture in a large mixing bowl. Sprinkle with cinnamon and stir to combine.

Meanwhile, melt virgin coconut oil and mix with maple syrup and vanilla extract. Pour virgin coconut oil syrup over oat mixture and stir to coat.

Spread evenly on a baking sheet and bake in oven for 10 minutes. Stir oat mixture and bake for another 5 minutes.

Remove from oven and pour mixture into a large glass bowl. Add chia seeds, raisins, and toasted coconut, and let cool.

Store in an airtight container and serve with almond milk or organic yogurt.

simple smoothie bowl

Serves 2

Add frozen cherries, frozen banana, dates, cashew butter and ¼ cup coconut water to a blender or food processor and blend to mix. Use more coconut water for a thinner consistency.

Add mixture to a deep bowl and top with cacao nibs, blueberries, shredded coconut, and your favorite granola.

2 cups frozen sweet dark cherries

1 frozen banana, sliced

4 pitted dates, chopped

¼ cup cashew butter

¼- ½ cup coconut water

2 tablespoons cacao nibs

¼ cup blueberries

2 tablespoons shredded coconut

½ cup granola (see page 32 & 34)

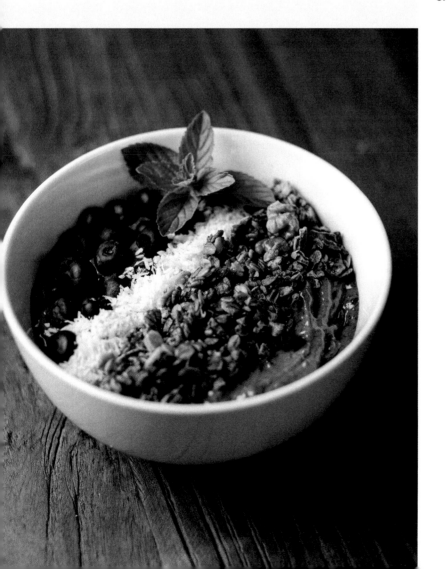

jackson hole zucchini muffins

Makes 12 large muffins

¼ cup golden flaxseeds, ground

3 cups organic unbleached white flour

1 tablespoon cinnamon

1 teaspoon nutmeg (may add more if desired)

2 teaspoons baking soda

½ teaspoon sea salt

3 cups zucchini, grated

1 cup organic cane sugar

1 tablespoon vanilla extract

¾ cup organic virgin coconut oil, melted

½ cup raisins

¼ cup dried cherries

½ cup walnuts

½ cup unsweetened shredded coconut

Preheat oven to 350°F.

Spray large muffin tray with cooking spray.

In a small bowl, combine ground flaxseeds and ½ cup water. Stir to mix and let sit for 10 minutes or until mixture forms a pudding consistency. (This combination can be used in place of 2 eggs)

Meanwhile, in a medium bowl combine flour, cinnamon, nutmeg, and baking soda and mix well.

In another medium size bowl combine zucchini, sugar, vanilla, coconut oil and flaxseed water mixture. Mix well.

Add in flour mixture and stir to combine.

Mix in raisins, dried cherries, walnuts, and coconut.

Using two large spoons, add batter to muffin tray filling each muffin hole completely to the top. Drizzle tops with honey and a sprinkle of brown sugar.

Bake for 18-20 minutes or until toothpick inserted comes out clean.

Let sit for 20 minutes before removing from muffin tray. Use a knife to cut around edges of each muffin to remove. Store in a large plastic container.

kristen:
This recipe was created in Jackson Hole while I was asked to whip up something to serve for my best friend's pre-wedding brunch using only the items I could find in her cupboard. Sometimes everything but the kitchen sink makes the best recipe. They were a total hit and the wedding was perfect.

flax bran muffins

Serves 12

Preheat oven to 350°F.

Combine flour, flaxseeds, oat bran, sugar, agave, baking soda, baking powder, salt, and cinnamon in a large bowl and mix well.

Use a cheese grater to shred carrots and apples. Add carrots, apples, raisins, and nuts.

In a separate bowl, blend egg whites, milk, and vanilla.

Add liquid ingredients to dry ingredients; mix until just combined. Do not over stir.

Coat muffin tin with virgin coconut oil. Divide mixture into 12 muffin cups.

Bake for 25-28 minutes. Allow to cool slightly; remove from muffin tin to finish cooling.

tip ▶ Make your own oat bran to use in baking by simply blending rolled oats in a food processor.

1½ cups white whole wheat flour

¾ cup ground flaxseeds

¾ cup oat bran (use rolled oats and blend in coffee grinder or food processor)

½ cup brown sugar + 1 tablespoon agave nectar

2 teaspoons baking soda

1 teaspoon baking powder

½ teaspoon sea salt

2 teaspoons cinnamon

1½ cups carrots, shredded

2 medium apples, unpeeled, shredded

½ cup raisins

¾ cup chopped walnuts, toasted

3 egg whites (free-range)

¾ cup almond milk

1 teaspoon vanilla extract

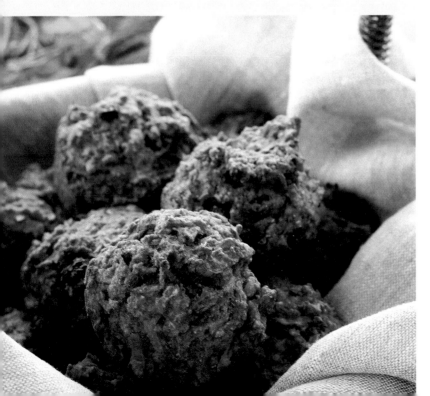

pumpkin apple muffins

2 cups almond flour

2 cups rolled oats

1 teaspoon baking soda

1 tablespoon pumpkin pie spice

½ teaspoon sea salt

1/3 cup virgin coconut oil, melted

3/4 cup maple syrup

2 tablespoons apple cider vinegar

1 tablespoon vanilla extract

1 cup pumpkin puree

2 organic cage-free eggs

2 Gala apples, chopped

¼ cup organic brown sugar (for topping)

Makes 10 large muffins

Preheat oven to 350° F.

Grease a muffin pan with virgin coconut oil spray.

Combine all ingredients besides brown sugar in a large bowl and mix well with a large spoon or with a hand-held beater. Add large spoonfuls of batter to muffin tin.

Sprinkle tops with a little bit of brown sugar and bake for 20-25 minutes or until toothpick comes out clean.

oatmeal pancakes

Serves 4 (Makes about 10 pancakes)

Mix all ingredients except oil in a blender until smooth (add more milk for creamier batter).

Pour into large bowl; let stand for 5 minutes.

Pour ⅓ cup batter per pancake onto hot, oiled griddle. Cook until bubbles form, then flip.

Serve topped with a spoonful of fruit, natural applesauce, or pure maple syrup.

2 tablespoons almond or coconut milk

5 egg whites

2 large eggs

1½ cups rolled oats

½ cup low-fat cottage cheese

½ cup natural unsweetened applesauce

½ teaspoon vanilla extract

½ teaspoon cinnamon

½ tablespoon virgin coconut oil

matt: *My childhood memories recall weekend breakfasts which always included these pancakes. They were Dad's creation. He always made them on Mother's Day. Guests are always surprised to find out the ingredients. I like to add sliced banana or blueberries to the batter. Oh...and if you haven't done it before, breakfast for dinner is Target to Table approved.*

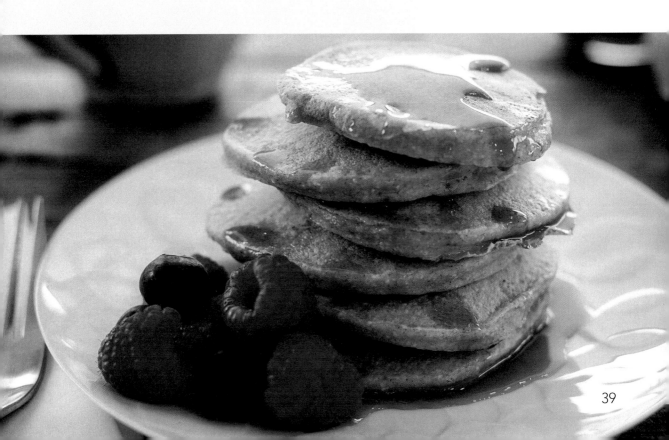

smoky salmon hash

Serves 4-6

Preheat oven to 350°F.

1 (2-pound) salmon fillet, with the skin on

Extra virgin olive oil

6 redskin potatoes, rinsed in water and diced

Sea salt & black pepper

1 large onion, thinly sliced

1 medium red bell pepper, thinly sliced

1 medium yellow bell pepper, thinly sliced

1 small green pepper, thinly sliced

2 cloves garlic, minced

2 green onions, finely chopped

3 sprigs fresh thyme, chopped

1 teaspoon smoked paprika

Pinch cayenne pepper

White vinegar

4 to 6 large eggs

Place the salmon on a large baking sheet skin-side down. Drizzle salmon with extra virgin olive oil and season with salt and black pepper to taste. Place into the oven and bake for 30 minutes until flaky. Remove from oven and set aside.

Add 2 tablespoons extra virgin olive oil to a large sauté pan over medium-high heat. Add the potatoes and sprinkle with salt and black pepper. Brown on all sides until tender. Transfer potatoes to a large serving bowl.

Add another 2 tablespoons extra virgin olive oil to the sauté pan, and sauté the onions, peppers, garlic, and thyme over medium-high heat. Season with salt, black pepper, smoked paprika, and cayenne pepper and cook until vegetables are tender.

Remove salmon from skin, and crumble it into the hash mixture. Cover to keep warm while you poach the eggs.

To poach eggs, place a large sauté pan over medium heat and fill with a few inches of water. Heat until it simmers. Add a splash of white vinegar. Using a wooden spoon, stir the water in one direction to create a small whirlpool. Add the eggs, one at a time, to the swirling water. Poach to desired doneness. Remove with a slotted spoon.

Serve the poached eggs on top of the hash mixture.

matt: *This dish is our family brunch staple.*

tip ▶ The salmon and potato mixture can be made ahead the day before and reheated in the oven when ready to serve with fresh eggs.

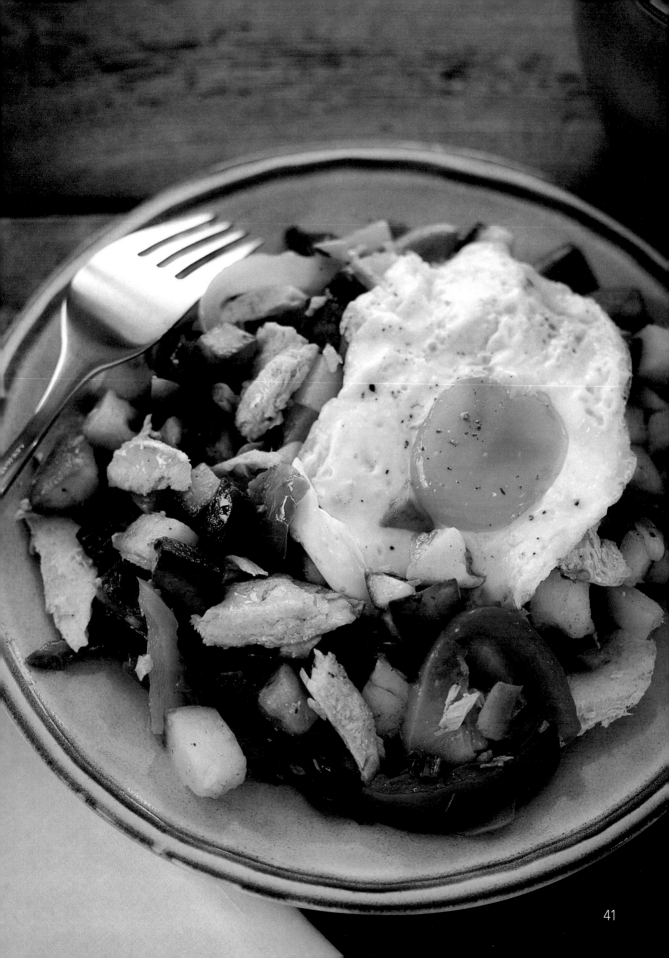

For the crust
(see recipe on page 44)

7 large eggs

½ cup unsweetened coconut milk or milk of choice

½ teaspoon sea salt

¼ teaspoon black pepper

1 cup spinach, chopped

1 tomato, seeds removed and diced

4 ounces feta cheese, crumbled

spinach & feta quiche

Serves 8

Preheat oven to 350°F.

In a large bowl whisk the eggs and milk to combine. Add salt and black pepper, then add the vegetables and feta cheese. Pour the egg mixture into baked pie crust.

Bake for 45-60 minutes or until fork comes out clean. Let sit 5 minutes before serving.

tip▶ Adding coconut milk makes the eggs nice and fluffy.

For the crust
(see recipe on page 44)

7 large eggs

½ cup unsweetened coconut milk or milk of choice

½ teaspoon sea salt

¼ teaspoon black pepper

1 10-ounce package California style frozen vegetables, thawed (carrots, cauliflower, zucchini, broccoli)

¼ cup green onions

2 nitrate-free sweet Italian chicken sausages, diced

½ cup raw milk cheddar cheese, shredded

chicken sausage & veggie pie

Serves 8

Preheat oven to 350°F.

In a large bowl whisk the eggs and milk to combine. Add salt and black pepper, then add the vegetables, sausage and cheese. Pour the egg mixture into baked pie shells.

Bake for 45-60 minutes or until fork comes out clean. Let sit 5 minutes before serving.

tip▶ May use organic frozen pie shells if not making Oatmeal Pie Crust

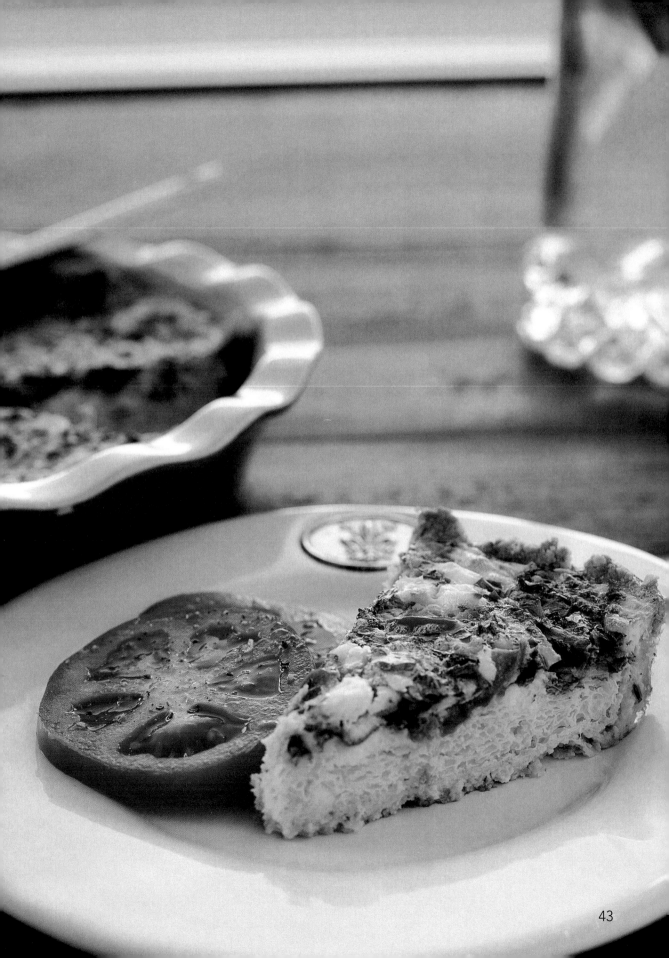

43

oatmeal raisin scones

Makes 8-9 large scones

1 ¼ cups organic unbleached white flour

1 ¼ cups rolled oats

1 ½ teaspoons aluminum free baking powder

¼ teaspoon food grade baking soda

¼ teaspoon sea salt

½ cup chopped pecans

½ cup golden raisins

1 teaspoon ground cinnamon

¼ cup cold unsalted butter, cut into pieces (about ¼ stick)

½ cup maple syrup

1 teaspoon pure vanilla extract

½ cup organic whipping cream or coconut milk

1 egg

Maple Syrup Glaze

1 cup organic powdered sugar

2 tablespoons maple syrup

2 tablespoons water

Preheat oven to 350° F.

Add all ingredients to a large mixing bowl except for the maple syrup, vanilla extract, cream or milk, and egg and mix well with a large spoon.

In a separate bowl, combine maple syrup, vanilla extract cream or milk and egg and mix well with a whisk. Add wet ingredients to dry ingredients and mix well.

Using a large spoon, drop batter onto a non-stick baking sheet. (May use parchment paper to prevent sticking.) The batter should make about 8-9 large scones.

Bake for 30-35 minutes or until dough is cooked through. Meanwhile, combine glaze ingredients in a small bowl and mix well.

Remove scones from oven and let cool before drizzling with glaze.

tip ▶ To make scones ahead of time, simply freeze the spooned-out dough on a waxed paper-lined baking sheet and place in the freezer for at least 4 hours or overnight. Once frozen, remove frozen dough from baking sheet and store in the freezer for 2-3 weeks. To bake, place frozen dough on a baking sheet and bake for 35-50 minutes. Glaze should be made fresh.

oatmeal pie crust

Makes one 9-inch crust

Preheat oven to 400°F. Coat a 9-inch pie dish with extra virgin olive oil.

Put the oats, flour, and salt in the bowl of a food processor and pulse to combine. Add the butter and pulse until you get a pebbly texture. Add the milk to combine.

Form the mixture into a ball and place between two sheets of floured waxed paper. Roll into a 10-inch circle. Remove the top sheet of waxed paper and flip the crust side onto the pie dish.

Gently remove the second layer of waxed paper, and press the crust into the corners of the dish. Fold over any crust that overlaps the edge of the dish.

Bake for 10 minutes and then remove to cool before adding egg mixture.

tip ▶ To save time in the kitchen, you may use a frozen organic pie crust from the grocery store.

¾ cup rolled oats

½ cup whole wheat flour

¼ teaspoon sea salt

3 tablespoons cold grass-fed butter, cut into small pieces

3 tablespoons coconut milk (or milk of choice)

asparagus & parmesan frittata

Serves 6-8

Preheat oven to 350°F.

Whisk all ingredients together in a mixing bowl.

Spray extra virgin olive oil on a mini muffin pan and fill each spot with the egg mixture.

Cook for 8-10 minutes or until cooked through. Serve immediately.

 These little bundles are light and fluffy. This is an elegant way to make a breakfast item that isn't full of high fat ingredients.

6 free-range eggs

1 cup almond or coconut milk

¼ cup fresh Parmesan cheese

½ cup small asparagus, chopped

½ teaspoon sea salt

¼ teaspoon black pepper

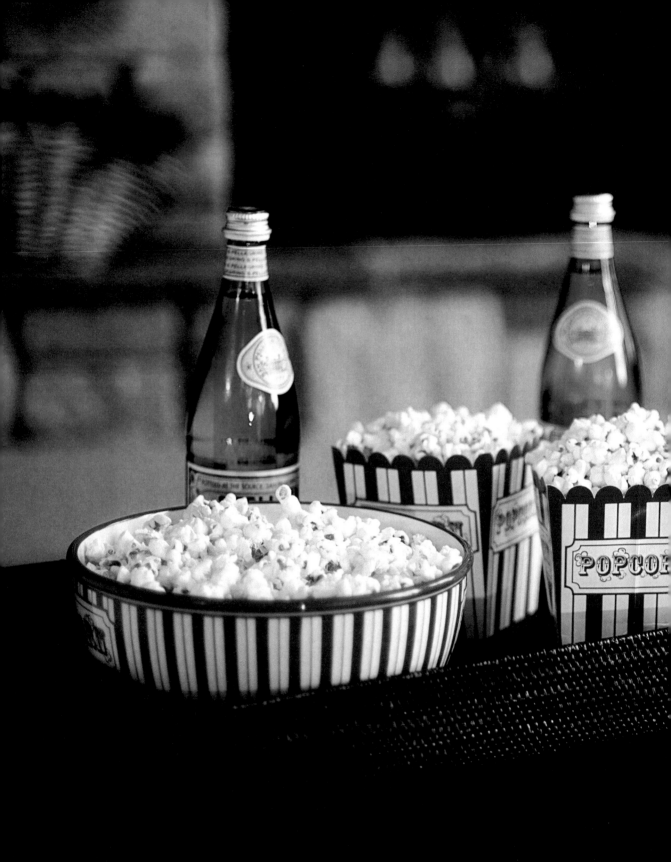

snacks

roasted spiced chickpeas

Serves 4

2 cans chickpeas

1 tablespoon extra virgin olive oil

1 teaspoon cumin

1 teaspoon chili powder

¼ teaspoon cayenne pepper

½ teaspoon sea salt

Preheat oven to 350°F.

Drain and rinse 2 cans of chickpeas and pat dry with paper towel.

Mix with 1 tablespoon extra virgin olive oil and spices.

Spread on parchment lined baking sheet and bake for 45-50 minutes, stirring frequently.

They will dry and become crunchy. Watch carefully so they don't burn.

kale chips

1 bunch kale, stems removed, then chopped

1 tablespoon extra virgin olive oil

Sea salt & black pepper to taste

Preheat oven to 350°F.

Toss kale with extra virgin olive oil, salt, and black pepper. Spread evenly in one layer on a large cookie sheet.

Place on middle rack in the oven.

Stir and flip frequently until the kale is crunchy and golden brown, approximately 20-25 min.

The kale will initially wilt, but will then start to dry and crisp. Watch carefully.

 This is a yummy guilt-free chip!

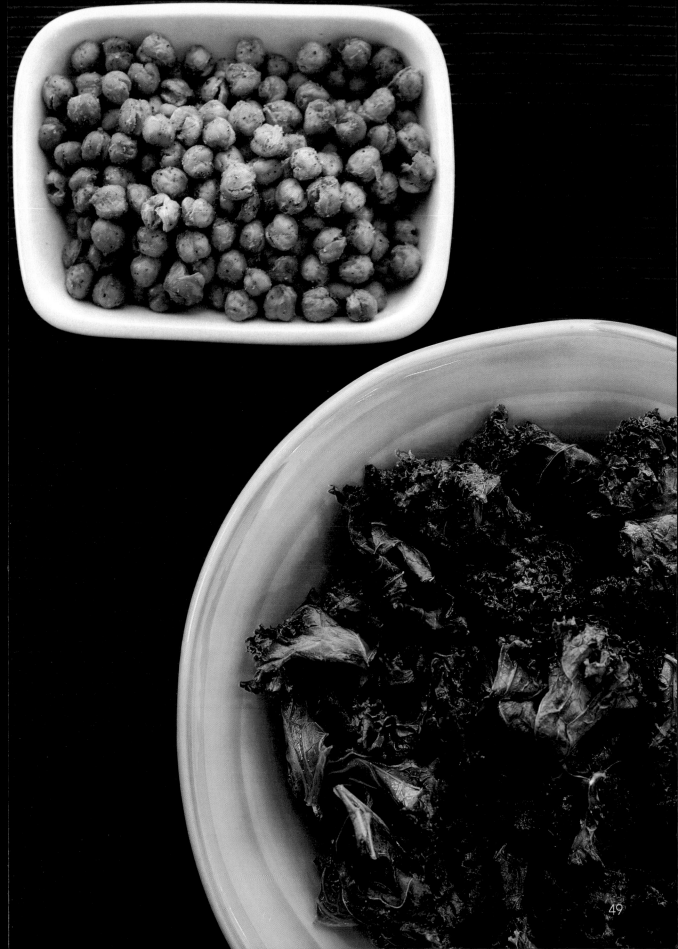

49

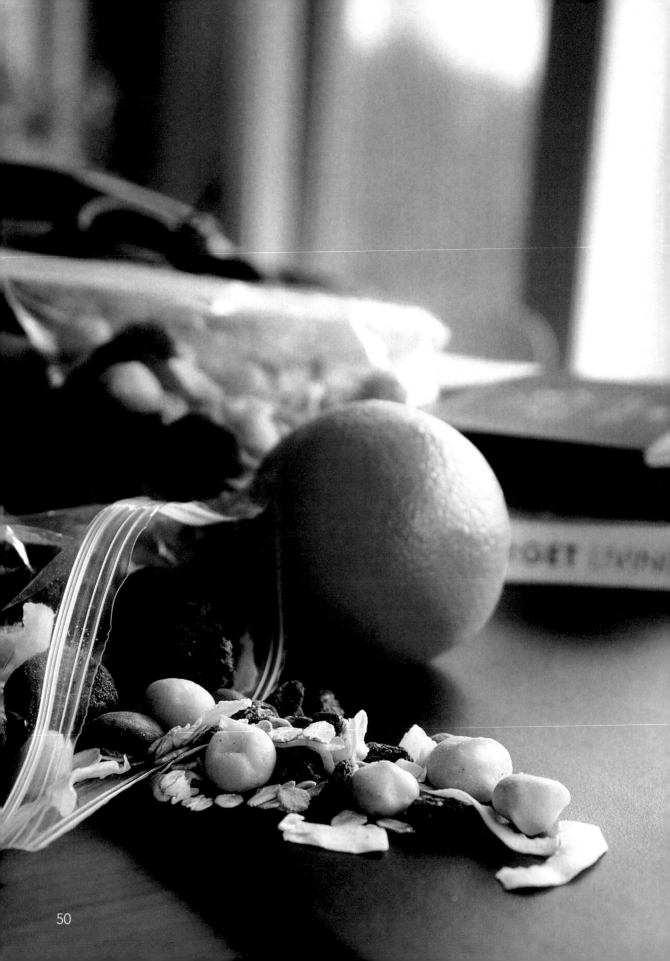

travel trail mix

Serves 2

Combine ingredients in a small sandwich bag to take on the go.

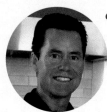

chris: *I created this snack out of desperation. I found myself stuck in the airport with very few healthy food options. If you find yourself sitting next to me on an airplane, I might share my stash with you.* ☺

1 tablespoon cacao nibs

2 Turkish figs

½ cup rolled oats

¼ cup raw macadamia nuts or nuts of choice

2 tablespoons raisins

2 tablespoons shredded coconut

coconut oil kettle corn

Serves 2

Heat coconut oil in saucepan. Drop 2 popcorn kernels in oil and wait until kernels pop. Once popped, add in the rest of the kernels and cover with a tight fitting lid.

Pop for 2-3 minutes or until the popping noise stops.

While popcorn is hot, stir in 1 tablespoon of agave nectar, a sprinkle of cinnamon, and sea salt to taste.

1 tablespoon virgin coconut oil

¼ cup popcorn kernels

1 tablespoon agave nectar

Cinnamon for sprinkling

Sea salt to taste

tip► Leave out the agave and cinnamon for a traditional popcorn taste.

 A healthy alternative to theatre-style popcorn.

honey flax energy bites

Makes 30

2 cups rolled oats

1 cup natural peanut butter

½ cup raw honey

1 cup ground flaxseeds

1 teaspoon vanilla extract

1 tablespoon virgin coconut oil

Optional add-ins:

 dark chocolate chips

 organic shredded coconut

 cacao nibs

Mix all ingredients together.

Coat hands with virgin coconut oil and form batter into small balls.

Store in refrigerator for 1 hour before serving. Freezes well.

 So amazingly delicious you may even reintroduce this recipe as a healthy dessert.

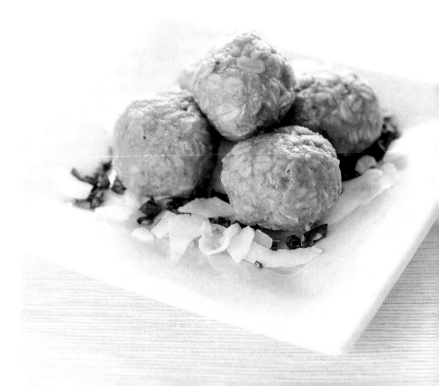

apricot almond coconut bars

Makes 8 (4-inch) bars

In a food processor, add apricots and blend until puréed.

Add in almond butter, rolled oats, coconut, and vanilla extract.

Blend until mixture forms a thick paste.

Place mixture in a small, square cake pan. Press to mold into pan.

Freeze for 20 minutes and cut into small bars.

Bars can be stored in the refrigerator for 1-2 weeks or in the freezer for up to 3 months.

1 12-ounce bag dried apricots

¾ cup almond butter

½ cup rolled oats

1 cup toasted raw coconut

1 tablespoon vanilla extract

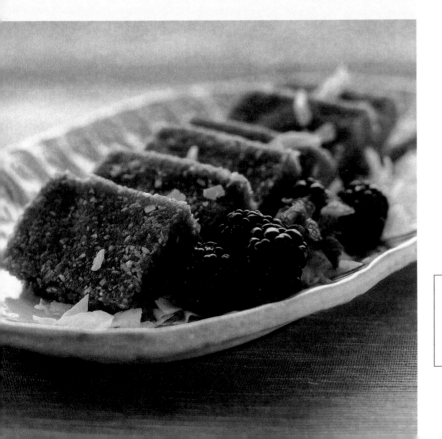

 This is a great alternative to the highly processed food bars found in most grocery stores.

53

homemade applesauce

Serves 4-6

3 pounds (10-12) small apples, cored and peeled

1 tablespoon ground cinnamon or 2 cinnamon sticks

1 teaspoon vanilla extract

Cut cored apples into large wedges and combine all ingredients in a large slow cooker. Cook on low for 4-6 hours or high for 2-3 hours.

"When life gives you apples, make applesauce."

 For added fiber, leave the skin on the apples

buffalo cauliflower

Serves 6

1 cup water

1 cup white whole wheat flour

½ teaspoon sea salt

1 tablespoon garlic powder

1 head of cauliflower, broken into small florets

1 bottle of hot sauce

1 tablespoon butter, melted

Preheat oven to 450°F.

Lightly spray a large nonstick baking sheet with oil.

Combine water, flour, salt, and garlic powder in a large bowl, and stir until well mixed.

Add the cauliflower pieces to the flour mixture and coat well.

Transfer coated cauliflower to baking sheet and bake for 20 minutes.

Meanwhile, combine the hot sauce and butter in a small bowl.

Pour hot sauce mixture over the baked cauliflower and continue baking for another 5 minutes.

Serve with your favorite ranch dressing or blue cheese dip and celery sticks for a guilt-free tailgate dish!

tip ▶ See Ranch Dressing recipe, page 98.

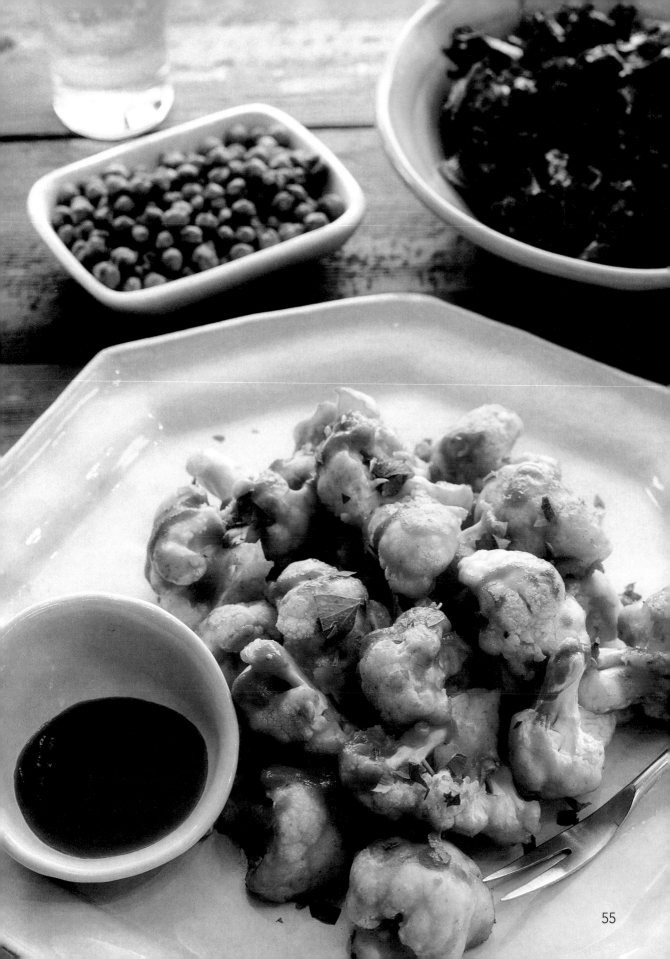

55

sean's guaca-money

Serves 6

3 avocados

½ cup sweet onions, chopped

1 cup tomatoes, chopped

Juice of 1 lime

½ teaspoon sea salt

½ teaspoon pepper

2 cloves garlic, minced (optional)

1 bunch cilantro, finely chopped (optional)

Peel and chop avocado, and place in large mixing bowl.

Crush avocados with a fork.

Add in the remaining ingredients and mix to combine.

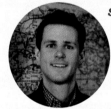

sean: I won Kristen's heart with this money recipe.

bomb diggity salsa

Makes about 6 cups

½ small Vidalia onion, finely chopped

½ pint multi-color cherry tomatoes, sliced

½ jalapeno seeds removed and diced

½ cup of fresh cilantro

Salt to taste

Combine all ingredients in a food processor and blend to mix until colorful but still a little chunky.

Serve with tortilla chips, chicken, steak, seafood, eggs, or refried beans and rice.

greek layer dip

Serves 4-6

Heat a large skillet over medium-high heat and add in one tablespoon extra virgin olive oil. Add ground meat and seasoning and cook until browned.

In a casserole dish or glass trifle dish, spread each ingredient in a single layer starting with hummus, ground meat, red onion, tzatziki sauce, cucumbers, yellow peppers, tomatoes, olives, feta and parsley.

Serve immediately or refrigerate until read to eat.

Serve with pita chips.

tip ▶ To make tzatziki sauce combine 1 cup of organic Greek yogurt, 1 teaspoon garlic powder, 1 teaspoon onion powder, ½ teaspoon salt, 1 tablespoon dried or fresh mint leaves or dill, and ½ lemon, juiced in a small bowl and mix well.

1 pound ground lamb or grass- fed beef

1 tablespoon herbes de Provence or Greek seasoning

1 teaspoon garlic powder

½ teaspoon cinnamon

Sea salt and pepper to taste

1 cup hummus (see recipe page 122)

½ red onion, diced

1 cup tzatziki sauce (see tip)

½ cup cucumbers, diced

½ cup yellow peppers, chopped

½ cup tomatoes, diced

½ cup pitted Kalamata olives, chopped

½ cup feta cheese, crumbled

¼ cup fresh parsley, chopped

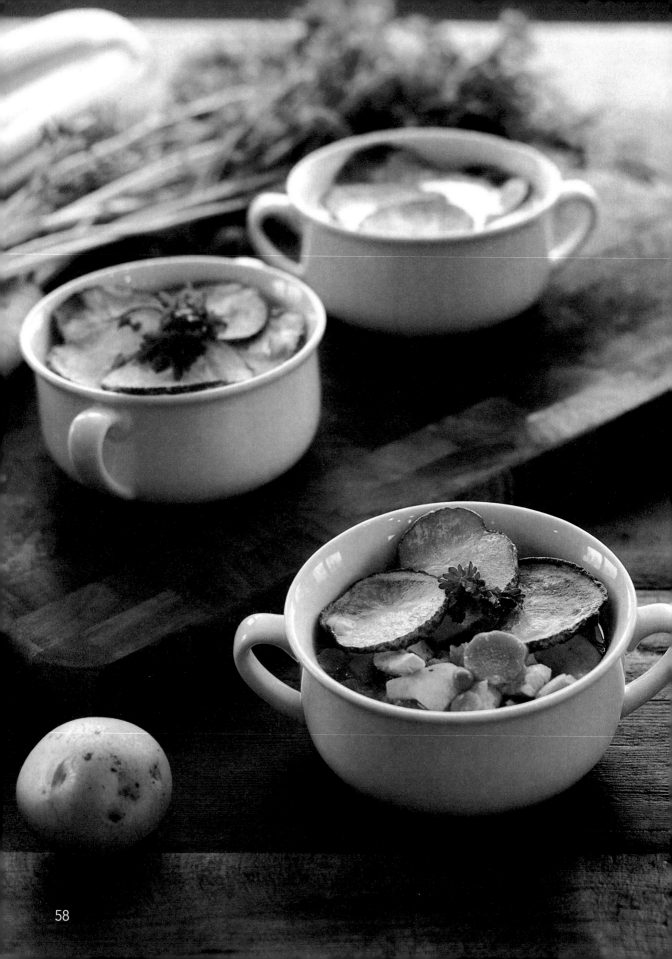

soups

chicken pot pie soup

Serves 4-6 (pictured on page 58)

For the soup:

2 tablespoons extra virgin olive oil

3 medium carrots, sliced

3 stalks celery, sliced

2-3 redskin potatoes, peeled and cubed

2 cups mushrooms, diced

2 cloves garlic, minced

½ large yellow onion, diced

2 chicken breasts, cubed

Sea salt & black pepper

Onion powder

Garlic powder

Dried thyme

¾ cup frozen peas

1 pack concentrated chicken stock or 1 tablespoon chicken soup base

16 ounces chicken stock

1 container organic cream of chicken soup

1 bay leaf

For the "crust:"

1 large russet potato, sliced thin with a mandolin (6 slices per serving bowl)

 When using store-bought soups, choose organic.

To make the soup:

In large Dutch oven, heat extra virgin olive oil over medium heat.

Add all the chopped vegetables except the frozen peas to the pan and cook for 2-3 minutes until the vegetables start to become tender.

Season the cubed chicken with garlic powder, sea salt, black pepper, onion powder, and thyme. Add the chicken to the vegetables in the pan and cook for another 5 minutes. Do not overcook the chicken as it will become dry.

Add the peas, concentrated chicken stock or soup base, and 16 ounces of chicken stock to the pot.

Add 1 teaspoon of thyme, bay leaf and 1 tablespoon of sea salt, and cook over medium low heat uncovered for 30 minutes.

After 30 minutes, add the cream of chicken soup and stir. Heat for 3 minutes on medium heat and let cool to serving temperature.

To make the "crust:"

Potato slices serve as the upper crust. While everything is cooking, thinly slice the russet potato. You will need about 6 slices per individual serving.

Lightly oil a large sheet pan. Lay the slices of potato in a pinwheel pattern. Repeat for as many individuals you plan to serve. Sprinkle the tops of the potato pinwheels with extra virgin olive oil and season with salt and black pepper. Bake in 350°F oven for about 30 minutes until lightly browned.

Serve in individual bowls and top with potato pinwheels.

south of the border chicken corn chowder

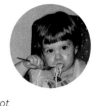

matt: I made this soup for the family and forgot to remove the jalapeño seeds. Needless to say, they were pretty hot under the collar.

Serves 6

Place chicken and celery in a medium sauce pan. Fill with enough water to cover chicken. Add ½ teaspoon sea salt. Cook for 20-25 minutes. Remove chicken from broth to cool. Using two forks, pull chicken apart into bite-size pieces.

Meanwhile, boil cubed potatoes in a separate pot until al dente. Remove from water and set aside.

Turn oven on high broil. Slice 2 of the Roma tomatoes in half lengthwise. Place the tomatoes and peppers in a single layer on ½ of a large baking sheet. Place 2 cups of corn on the remaining half of baking sheet. Drizzle with extra virgin olive oil and season with sea salt and black pepper. Broil for 10 minutes then turn the tomatoes and peppers, and toss the corn. Return to broil for another 10 more minutes, watching carefully not to burn the vegetables but allowing them to get a slight char.

Once cooled, remove the skin of the tomatoes. Set aside one cup roasted corn for later.

Place 1 cup of the chicken broth, roasted tomatoes, peppers, and 1 cup of corn into the blender. Blend for 10-15 seconds.

In Dutch oven heat 1 tablespoon of extra virgin olive oil over medium heat. Add onions and garlic, and cook for 3 minutes. Add the pulled chicken, onion powder and sriracha chili sauce. Cook for 3 minutes. Add 2 cups chicken broth and continue to cook for 5 minutes. Add the blended liquid, potatoes, and reserved roasted corn. Chop the remaining 2 Roma tomatoes and add them to the soup. Cover the soup and simmer for 20 minutes.

Serve with sliced avocado and tortilla chips on top.

2 boneless, skinless chicken breasts

3 celery stalks

½ teaspoon sea salt

1½ cups cubed potatoes, skin on

4 Roma tomatoes

1 red pepper, washed and quartered

1 green pepper, washed and quartered

½ jalapeño, sliced lengthwise and seeds removed

2 cups frozen corn, thawed

3 cups chicken broth

½ yellow onion, diced

3 cloves of garlic, diced

2 teaspoons sriracha chili sauce

1 teaspoon onion powder

Extra virgin olive oil

Sea salt & black pepper to taste

Garnish with sliced avocado and blue corn tortilla chips

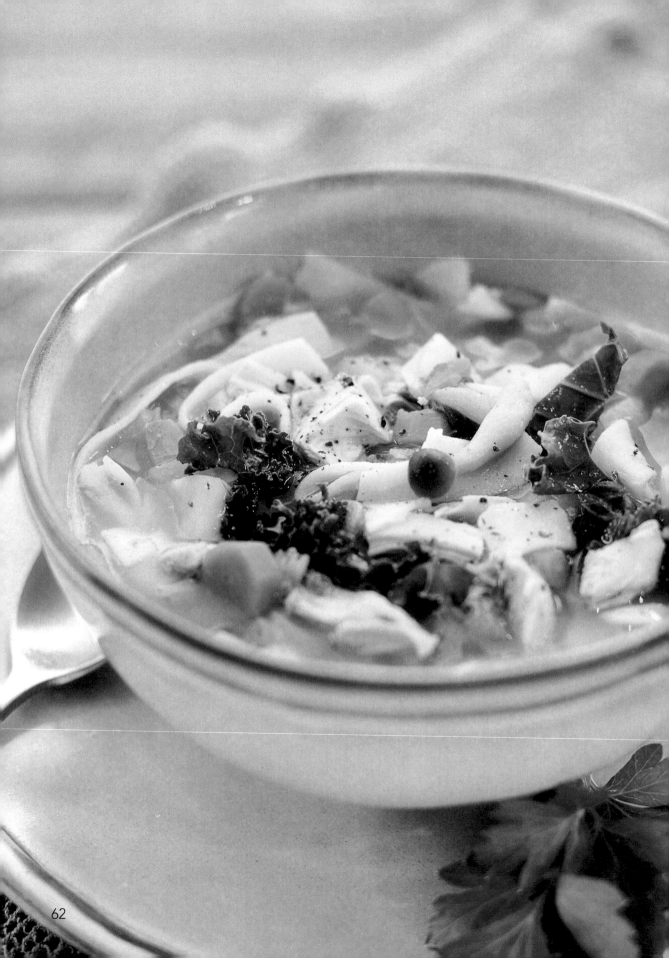

mom's chicken noodle soup

Serves 10-12

Clean chicken and place it whole in an 8-quart soup pot. Cover with fresh water. Add whole carrots, celery, 2 onions, sea salt, peppercorns, bay leaf, whole allspice, and stick cinnamon. Bring to a boil and then lower heat to simmer gently for 1 hour, until chicken is tender and broth is developed.

Remove chicken and set aside to cool. Strain broth, clean soup pot, and return strained broth to pot. Taste broth to determine if additional sea salt and/or black pepper is necessary and add to taste.

Add remaining vegetables except spinach or kale to the broth in the pot. Gently simmer for 20-30 minutes until vegetables are tender.

Meanwhile, cook pasta or rice, drain, and set aside.

After the vegetables in the broth are tender, add spinach or kale and simmer an additional 5 minutes.

Remove skin from chicken and chicken from the bone. Cut chicken into bite-sized pieces and return all the chicken to the soup pot. Add pasta or rice and heat for another 10 minutes.

Enjoy!

paula: *I was honored that my kids asked me to put my chicken soup recipe in their cookbook. Actually, this is my mom's chicken soup recipe, but we all love it. What hits the spot better than a bowl of homemade chicken noodle soup?*

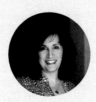

For the broth:

1 whole chicken (3-4 pounds)

2 whole carrots

2 stalks celery with leaves

2 small-sized onions, peeled, whole

2 tablespoons coarse sea salt

1 tablespoon whole peppercorns

1 bay leaf

1 tablespoon whole allspice

2 sticks cinnamon

For the soup:

2 cups carrots, chopped

2 cups celery, chopped

1 pound mushrooms, sliced

6 small-sized onions, peeled, left whole

4 cups cooked egg noodles (or your favorite pasta or rice)

2 cups baby spinach or chopped kale

tip ▶ Cinnamon and allspice are the secret ingredients that make this soup taste like mom's.

wild rice soup with mushrooms & pesto

Serves 6-8

For the chicken stock:

1 whole chicken

5 large carrots, washed not peeled, rough chopped in 3-inch pieces

5 large celery stalks washed, rough chopped in 3-inch pieces

1 large onion, washed not peeled, cut into 4 pieces

1 tablespoon peppercorns

2 tablespoons sea salt

10 stalks thyme

1 large stalk rosemary

Handful fresh parsley

For the soup:

3 large carrots, peeled and sliced

1 pint mushrooms, sliced

2 cups cooked wild rice

2 cups baby spinach

For the pesto:

1 cup walnuts

4 cups fresh basil

1 cup spinach

2 tablespoons extra virgin olive oil

3 cloves garlic

1 teaspoon sea salt

To make the chicken stock:

Place all the ingredients in a large pot and fill with water (2 inches above the ingredients).

Bring to a boil and simmer for 1-2 hours or until the broth is golden and the chicken is cooked.

Strain the broth into a large soup pot.

Dispose of the veggies and set chicken aside.

Add the carrots and mushrooms to the pot of fresh chicken broth. Cook until vegetables are tender.

Add the cooked rice and spinach, and continue to cook until rice is warm and spinach is wilted.

Meanwhile, remove the skin from the chicken and remove all of the meat. Cut it into bite size pieces and toss into soup.

To make pesto:

Put all the pesto ingredients except the oil in a food processor, start the food processor, and then drizzle in the oil until well combined.

Add the pesto to the soup. Season with additional sea salt and black pepper to taste and serve.

tip▶ This chicken stock can be made in advance and frozen for any recipe that calls for chicken stock. The chicken can be used for other recipes like the Awesome Chicken Salad on page 108.

64

white bean chicken chili

Serves 4

Cut chicken into bite sized pieces and season with salt and black pepper.

Heat oil in a large saucepan over medium-high heat. Add chicken and heat until cooked through and juices run clear.

Add in beans, salsa, and broth. Cook until heated through.

Sprinkle with cheese and top with crumbled tortilla chips.

Serve and enjoy while you watch your favorite game, movie or show.

1 pound boneless, skinless chicken breasts

1 tablespoon extra virgin olive oil

1 48-ounce jar great northern beans, drained and rinsed

1 24-ounce jar corn and black bean salsa

2 cups chicken broth

1 cup of shredded cheddar cheese

Organic tortilla chips for topping

Garnish with 1 cup shredded cheddar cheese and 2 cups crumbled blue corn chips

kristen: This was a staple meal when I was a broke college student living with 8 girls at WMU! Go Broncos!

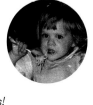

tip ▶ This recipe doubles and freezes well. To make this as a dip, simply leave out the chicken broth and serve with organic tortilla chips.

cook-off chili

Serves 4-6

10 ounces ground bison or turkey

1 cup onion, chopped

1 cup green pepper, chopped

2 teaspoons garlic, minced

1 15-ounce can kidney, black, or pinto beans, rinsed and drained

1 14.5-ounce can stewed tomatoes

1 8-ounce can tomato sauce

1 cup beef, chicken, or vegetable broth

½ cup filtered water

½ cup frozen corn

½ tablespoon chili powder

½ teaspoon cumin

½ teaspoon dried oregano

1 teaspoon fresh cilantro

Sea salt & black pepper, to taste

Garnish with avocado, onion, tomato, and/or cheese

Heat extra virgin olive oil in a 4-quart sauce pan over medium heat.

Brown ground meat in sauce pan.

Add onions, green pepper, and garlic. Heat until vegetables are tender and slightly browned.

Add remaining ingredients and simmer for 30 minutes.

Sprinkle with chopped avocado, onion, tomato, and/or cheese to serve.

tip▶ Can be made a day ahead and can be frozen for up to 3 months.

 A big part of our On Target Living program is teaching people how to feel and perform their best in work and in life. We conduct live, multi-day retreats that immerse attendees into the program. One of our retreat events is a team chili cook-off. Teams combine ingredients and flavors to make their own signature chili recipe. Judges choose the winners on taste, appearance, and creativity.

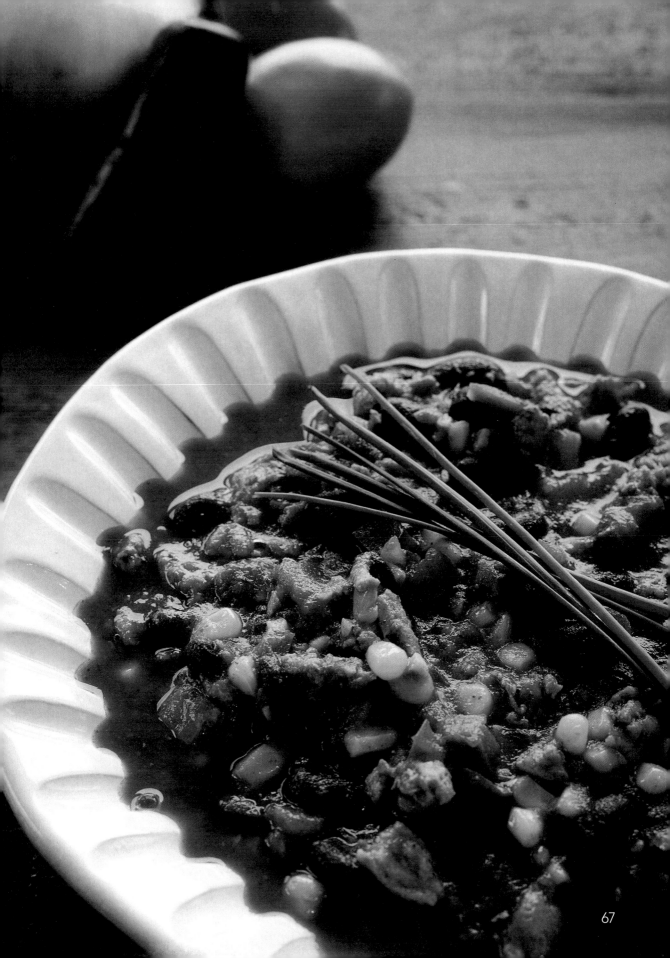

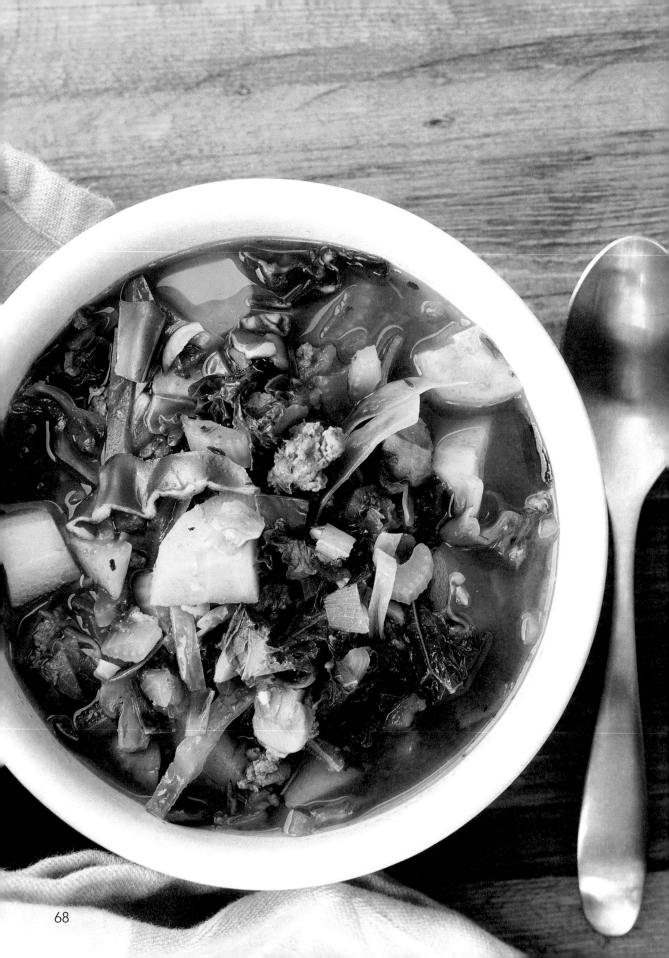

bison stew

Serves 6

Heat extra virgin olive oil over medium-high heat in a 6-quart saucepan.

Brown bison, then add onion and garlic, and cook until onions are soft.

Add remaining ingredients and simmer for 30 minutes or until vegetables are tender.

Let sit 10 minutes before serving.

Season with sea salt and black pepper to taste.

1 tablespoon extra virgin olive oil

1 pound ground bison

1 onion, chopped

3 cloves garlic, diced

1 tablespoon herbes de Provence

4 stalks celery, chopped

3 large parsnips, peeled and chopped

3 large carrots, peeled and chopped

1 pound button mushrooms, sliced

1 can Italian seasoned diced tomatoes

2 quarts chicken broth

½ head cabbage, sliced

2 cups kale, chopped

Sea salt & black pepper to taste

 Wild game, such as rabbit, pheasant, goose, duck, deer, bear, elk, and bison, consume a more natural diet. Their meat tends to have a lower fat content and contain more anti-inflammatory omega-3s than conventional meats.

italian zuppa

Serves 4-6

1 pound sweet Italian sausage

3 slices nitrate-free organic bacon

1 tablespoon Italian seasoning

1 onion, diced

2 cloves garlic, minced

7 cups chicken broth

1 cup water

4 large yellow potatoes, cut in half lengthwise and sliced thin

2 cups kale, chopped

Pinch of red pepper

Sea salt & black pepper to taste

½ cup organic half and half

Heat a large soup pot on medium-high heat.

Add sausage and bacon, and cook until sausage is cooked through and bacon is crispy.

Add Italian seasoning and stir to mix.

Add in onion and garlic, and cook until tender.

Add broth and water, and bring to a boil.

Add in sliced potatoes, and cook over medium heat for 5-10 minutes or until potatoes are al dente.

Add in kale, red pepper, and sea salt and black pepper to taste.

Turn off heat and stir in half and half.

Serve hot with fresh baked bread and parmesan cheese.

kristen: I owe this creation to the influence of my BFF Annie. We have so many memories and delicious creations from our days in the Johnson kitchen.

tomato basil soup

Serves 4-6

Heat extra virgin olive oil in a heavy-bottomed soup pot.

Sauté onion until soft and translucent, 3-5 minutes.

Add garlic and sauté until fragrant, 1 minute.

Add tomatoes, tomato paste, broth, dried basil, black pepper, and sea salt. Bring to a boil, reduce to a simmer and cook 10 minutes.

Stir in fresh basil and serve.

2 teaspoons extra virgin olive oil

1 medium onion, finely chopped

4 garlic cloves, minced

2 28-ounce cans crushed tomatoes

1 tablespoon tomato paste

2 ½ cups chicken broth

½ teaspoon dried basil

1 teaspoon coarse black pepper

2 teaspoons sea salt

20 leaves fresh basil, torn or coarsely chopped

very veggie soup

Serves 6-8

1 tablespoon extra virgin olive oil

1 yellow onion, chopped

3 cloves garlic, minced

1-inch fresh ginger, minced

2 cups celery, chopped

2 cups carrots, chopped

2 leeks, cleaned and chopped - using white parts only

5 sprigs fresh thyme

1 bay leaf

2 cups zucchini, diced

1 cup green cabbage, chopped

1 bunch Swiss chard or any greens of choice, stems remove and leaves chopped

8 cups vegetable broth

Heat oil in a large soup pot. Add in onion, garlic, ginger, celery, carrots, leeks, thyme, and bay leaf and simmer until vegetables are slightly tender, about 5 minutes. Season to taste with salt and black pepper.

Add in zucchini, cabbage, Swiss chard, and broth. Stir to mix and simmer for 10-15 minutes until vegetables are tender. Season again with salt and black pepper to taste.

tip ▶ To make it heartier, throw in cooked quinoa, farro, or any grain of choice.

 Give the body proper fuel, rest, and exercise, and it will naturally detoxify itself. There is no magic "juice" detox.

Chewing whole foods that are loaded with vitamins, minerals, antioxidants, protein, and fiber will help to stimulate digestive enzymes that assist with digestion and keep you feeling full and satisfied.

Why guzzle hundreds of calories worth of fruit when you can eat one serving of soup and actually feel full?

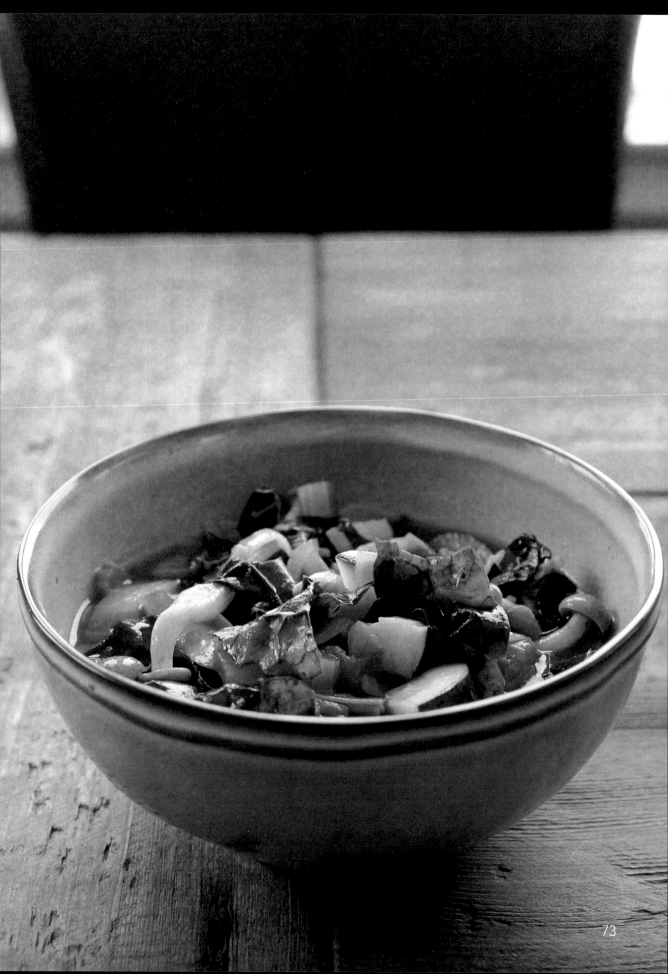

"fungi" mushroom soup

Serves 4

3 tablespoons extra virgin olive oil

10 ounces mushrooms of your choice, washed and chopped

1 yellow onion, chopped

2 garlic cloves, chopped

2 cups chicken broth

2 cups skim milk

8 ounces button mushrooms, washed and chopped

Sea salt & black pepper to taste

Garnish with fresh basil

Add 2 tablespoons extra virgin olive oil to a large soup pot. Sauté 10 ounces of mushrooms along with onions and garlic until the onions are translucent.

Add chicken broth and milk, and slowly bring to a boil. Cool for 5 minutes.

Carefully put all ingredients in blender and pulse for 30 seconds until puréed.

In a deep pan, sauté the button mushrooms in 1 tablespoon of extra virgin olive oil for 5 minutes.

Add the puréed soup.

Sprinkle with fresh basil.

 Mushrooms are high in energizing B vitamins and choline, which help fight inflammation. Mushrooms are also especially high in selenium, an antioxidant-rich mineral that helps strengthen the immune system and fight disease. Did you know that mushrooms are the only plant-based source of vitamin D?

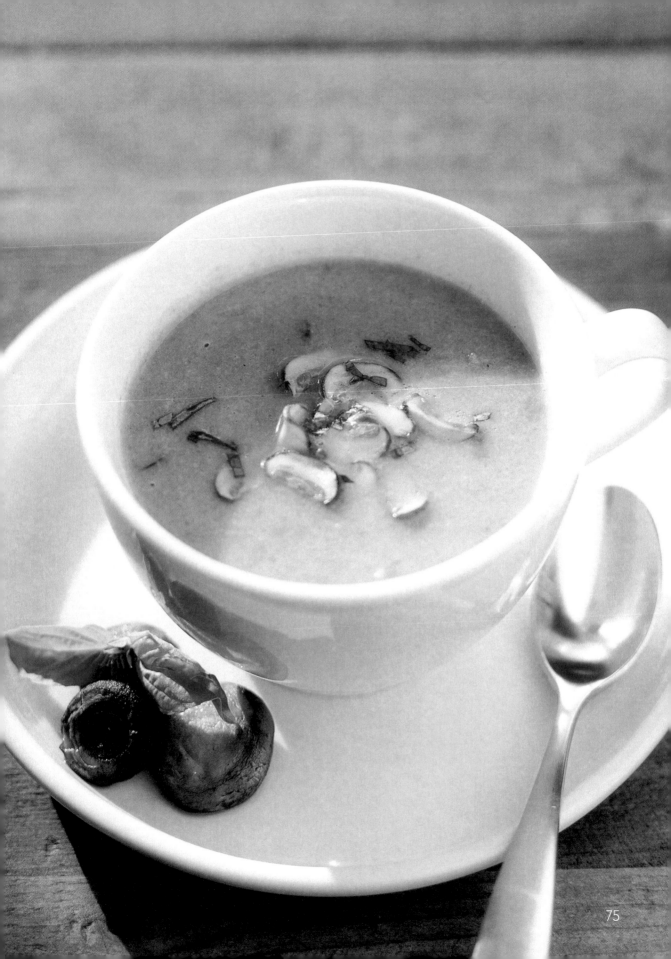

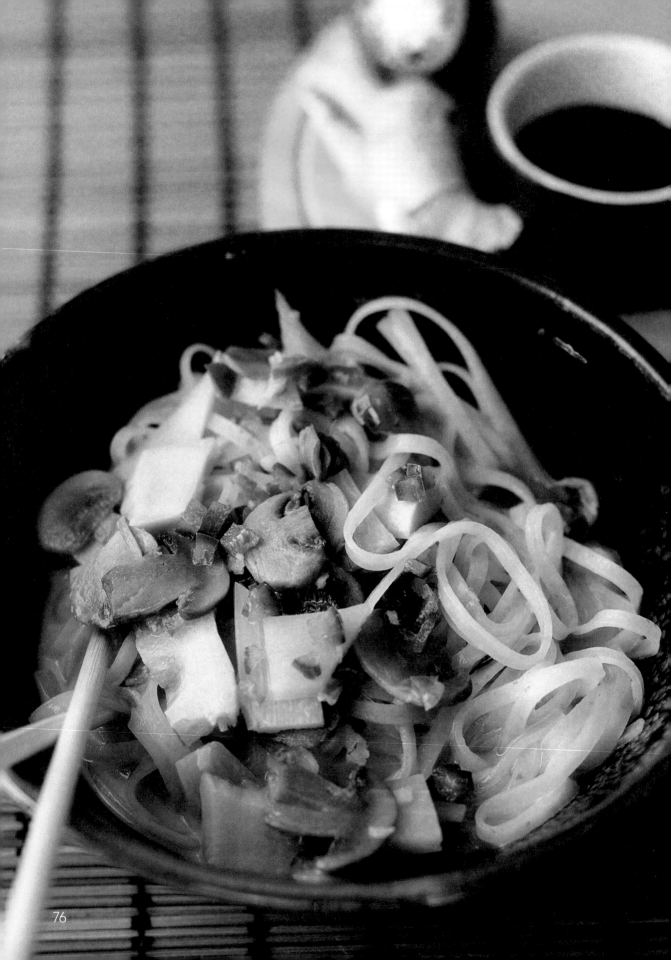

coconut ginger soup

Serves 4

In a small skillet cook mushrooms covered on medium-low heat until all the liquid has evaporated. Set aside.

In a large soup pot cook jalapeño and ginger in 1 tablespoon extra virgin olive oil over medium heat until tender.

Add in chicken broth, coconut milk, and Bragg's Liquid Aminos, and heat to a low boil. Do not over boil because the coconut milk will burn.

Add in ¾ of package of noodles and cook until al dente.

Add in reserved mushrooms, bamboo shoots, and green onions, and turn off heat.

Let soup sit for 5 minutes before serving.

Season with salt and black pepper to taste if needed. Top with fresh parsley.

Serve with a fork and a spoon.

1 pint mushrooms, sliced thin

1 small jalapeño pepper, seeds removed and diced

1 tablespoon ginger, grated with a microplane

1 quart chicken broth

1 can unsweetened coconut milk

⅓ cup Bragg's Liquid Aminos

1 package noodles (brown rice, soba, or udon)

1 small container bamboo shoots

½ cup green onions, sliced

Garnish with fresh parsley

This is a gourmet and healthy "ramen noodle soup."

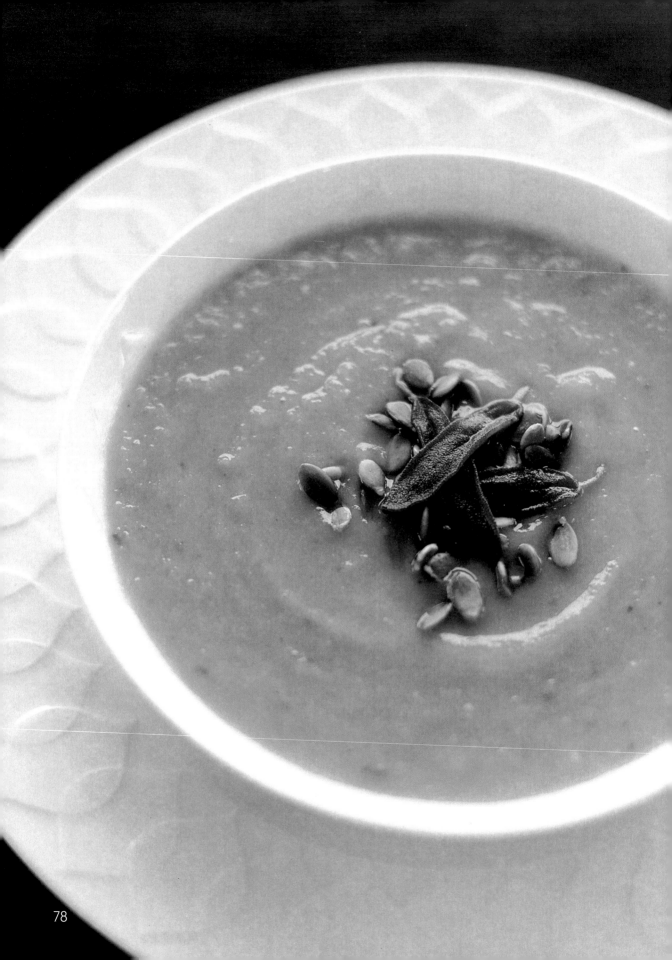

i love butternut squash soup

Serves 4-6

In an 8-quart soup pot, melt butter and oil together over medium-high heat. Add the onion, carrot, apple, and garlic, and sauté for about 5 minutes until the vegetables are soft.

Add the squash and the chicken stock. Bring mixture to a boil.

Add sage and lower to simmer for about 30 minutes until squash is tender.

Turn off the heat to cool slightly. Using a blender, food processor or immersion blender, blend the mixture until smooth and thick. Season with sea salt and black pepper.

Serve warm topped with toasted pumpkin seeds and fried sage leaves if desired.

2 tablespoons butter

2 tablespoons extra virgin olive oil

1 medium onion, chopped

1 medium carrot, peeled and chopped

1 medium apple, peeled and chopped

3 cloves garlic, minced

1 large butternut squash, peeled, seeded and cut into 1-inch pieces (about 8 cups)

6 cups chicken stock

Sea salt & black pepper to taste

¼ cup chopped fresh sage leaves

Garnish with ¼ cup toasted pumpkin seeds and 6 lightly fried fresh sage leaves

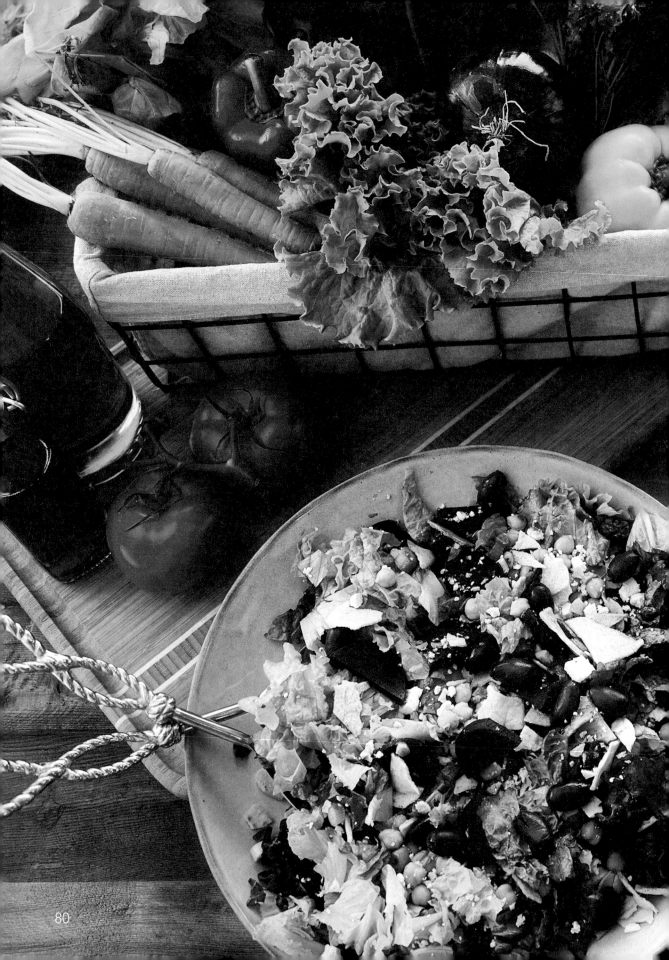

salads

dressings

mediterranean salad

Serves 4 (pictured on page 80)

Combine salad ingredients in a large bowl.

Toss with **Herb & Red Wine Vinaigrette** below.

Crumble toasted pita chips on top of salad for a little crunch.

1 small package baby spinach

2 heads romaine lettuce

1 can chickpeas, drained and rinsed

¼ cup feta cheese, crumbled

½ cup cherry tomatoes, halved

¼ cup pitted Kalamata olives or black olives

½ cup carrots, shredded

½ red onion, diced

1 large beet, boiled and sliced, or 1 can sliced beets

Pita chips

herb & red wine vinaigrette

Mix together dressing ingredients and toss into salad mixture.

½ cup red wine vinegar

½ cup extra virgin olive oil

1 teaspoon Dijon mustard

2 garlic cloves, diced

2 tablespoons fresh basil, chopped

1 tablespoon fresh parsley, chopped

¼ teaspoon honey

Sea salt & black pepper to taste

 Store-bought dressings can be expensive and unhealthy. Save money by making your own homemade versions with better ingredients.

taco salad

Serves 4

Brown ground meat in extra virgin olive oil over medium-high heat.

Add taco seasoning and water, and heat for 2 minutes or until liquid is absorbed.

Add the rest of the vegetable ingredients to the ground meat and toss into lettuce.

Toss with **Southwest Yogurt Dressing** below.

Top with cheese, salsa, guacamole, and crushed tortilla chips.

tip ▶ If you are short on time or want something easier, find an organic taco seasoning mix and use ½ packet for the meat mixture and ½ packet for the dressing.

Salad:

1 pound lean ground turkey, bison, or beef

1 tablespoon extra virgin olive oil

1 tablespoon Taco Seasoning (see recipe below)

¼ cup water

3 heads romaine lettuce, chopped

1 red bell pepper, chopped

1 small red onion, diced

1 can black beans, drained and rinsed

1 can corn, drained

Taco Seasoning:

1 tablespoon chili powder

1½ teaspoon cumin powder

¼ teaspoon garlic powder

¼ teaspoon onion powder

¼ teaspoon dried oregano

¼ teaspoon paprika

1 teaspoon sea salt

1 teaspoon black pepper

Pinch, cayenne pepper

southwest yogurt dressing

Combine dressing ingredients and toss into salad.

 Greek yogurt contains twice the protein of regular yogurt and less lactose.

1 6-ounce container plain Greek yogurt

¼ cup coconut milk

1 tablespoon Taco Seasoning

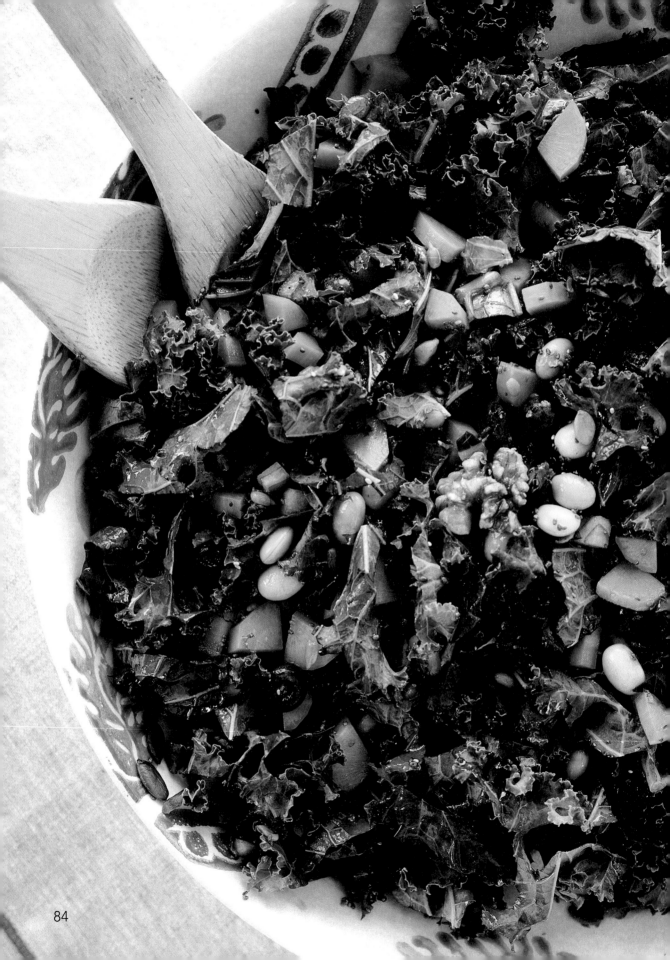

superfoods salad

Serves 6

Combine salad ingredients and toss in a large bowl.

Pour **Pomegranate Dressing** below over salad and toss to coat.

Refrigerate for 1 hour before serving.

Store in the refrigerator for up to 3 days.

1 bunch kale, stems removed and chopped

½ cup frozen, shelled edamame, thawed

1 pint blueberries, washed and drained

¼ cup pumpkin seeds

¼ cup walnuts, chopped

¼ cup goji berries

½ red onion, diced

3 large carrots, peeled and diced

2 tablespoons chia seeds

 Throw chia seeds and goji berries on top of a salad for a burst of flavor and nutrition.

pomegranate dressing

Combine dressing ingredients and mix well.

½ cup pure pomegranate juice

¼ cup extra virgin olive oil

1 tablespoon red wine vinegar

1 teaspoon ground turmeric

Sea salt & black pepper to taste

 Once in a while you can make Sunday a Salad Sunday night. It's a new way to reintroduce salads for dinner! After a long weekend of eating out and going out with friends, this may be exactly what you need to get back on your Target to Table track.

85

gyro greek salad

Serves 4

1 pound ground lamb, beef, or bison

2 tablespoons extra virgin olive oil

1 tablespoon Greek seasoning or ½ teaspoon dried oregano and ½ teaspoon dried mint

Sea salt and black pepper to taste

2 heads romaine lettuce, chopped

¼ cup pitted Kalamata olives

½ red onion, diced

1 small cucumber, peeled and diced

½ cup cherry tomatoes, halved

¼ cup feta cheese, crumbled

¼ cup pine nuts, toasted

Heat 1 tablespoon extra virgin olive oil in a large skillet over medium-high heat.

Cook ground meat and Greek seasoning until cooked through. Season with sea salt and black pepper.

Toss with **Greek Yogurt Dressing** below to coat.

Add remaining ingredients and top with ground meat and toasted pine nuts.

 Use extra virgin olive oil for cooking. Extra virgin means it is the first press of the olive retaining the most flavor and nutrition.

greek yogurt dressing

1 cup plain Greek yogurt

2 tablespoons red wine vinegar

1 tablespoon dried dill weed

1 tablespoon oregano

2 cloves garlic, minced

Sea salt & black pepper to taste

Combine dressing ingredients in a large bowl and stir to mix.

warm butternut & chickpea salad

Serves 4

Preheat oven to 425°F.

In large bowl, combine the butternut squash, garlic, olive oil, and a few pinches of sea salt. Toss the squash pieces until evenly coated.

Roast them on a baking sheet for 25 minutes, or until soft. Remove from the oven and cool.

To assemble the salad, combine the squash, chickpeas, onion, and cilantro or parsley in a large salad bowl.

Toss with **Tahini Dressing** below or serve dressing on the side.

Serve immediately.

1 medium butternut squash (2 to 2.5 pounds), peeled, seeded, and cut into 1½-inch pieces

1 medium garlic clove, minced or pressed

2 tablespoons extra virgin olive oil

Sea salt

1 15-ounce can chickpeas, drained and rinsed

¼ medium red onion, finely chopped

¼ cup fresh cilantro or parsley, chopped

tahini dressing

Combine the garlic and lemon juice in a small mixing bowl. Add the tahini and whisk to blend.

Gradually whisk in the olive oil and water until the dressing is combined. Add additional water to achieve desired consistency.

1 medium garlic clove, finely minced with a pinch of sea salt

¼ cup lemon juice

3 tablespoons tahini, well stirred

2 tablespoons water

2 tablespoons olive oil, plus more to taste

Tahini is a paste made from ground, hulled sesame seeds and used in North African, Greek, Turkish, and Middle Eastern cuisine. Tahini is a major component in hummus and baba ghanoush. It adds a creamy texture when used in salad dressings.

mexican kale salad

Serves 4

1 can vegetarian refried beans

1 bag tortilla chips

1 pound cheddar cheese, shredded

1 pound boneless, skinless chicken breasts

1 cup chicken broth

1 package taco seasoning (see page 83 for homemade Taco Seasoning recipe)

1 6-ounce package baby kale

½ cup green onions, chopped

½ cup frozen peas, thawed

¼ cup parmesan cheese, shredded

1 tomato, diced

Guacamole (see Guacamoney recipe on page 56)

 Remember to choose organic animal products (cheese, chicken, etc.) and organic corn products when available.

Preheat oven to 350°F.

Place refried beans in a small casserole dish and cover with foil. Place in oven to warm for 10-15 minutes.

Lay tortilla chips evenly on a large baking sheet. Using a spoon or spatula, spread warm refried beans on tortilla chips and top with cheddar cheese. Bake for 10-12 minutes or until cheese is melted.

Meanwhile, poach chicken breasts in chicken broth until tender. Leaving the chicken in the cooking liquid, set aside to cool slightly. Once chicken has cooled a bit, remove from liquid and shred by pulling meat apart with two forks.

Place shredded chicken in a skillet and add taco seasoning mixed with ¼ cup of warm water. Heat until chicken is warmed and liquid is absorbed, about 2-3 minutes.

For the salad, mix baby kale, green onions, peas, parmesan, tomatoes, and shredded chicken together in a large salad bowl. Toss with enough **Apple Cider Vinaigrette** below to coat the greens.

Remove tortilla chips from oven and evenly spread guacamole over chips.

Top tortilla chips with salad mixture and serve.

apple cider vinaigrette

1 cup raw apple cider vinegar

½ cup extra virgin olive oil

Sea salt & black pepper to taste

Whisk dressing ingredients and pour over salad (may not need all of dressing depending on the size of salad). Toss to mix.

rainbow ribbon salad

Serves 4

Peel sweet potatoes, carrots and beets. Using a potato peeler, slice lengthwise along sweet potato and carrots to form ribbon like strands. Do the same with the beets. If beets are small and hard to form ribbon like strands, use a mandolin and slice beets thinly. Add all peeled vegetables to a large mixing bowl.

Combine vinaigrette ingredients in a small food processor and blend to mix. Pour dressing over vegetables and toss to coat evenly.

Place dressed vegetables in a bowl. Seal and store in the refrigerator for two hours to marinate and soften vegetables before serving.

Remove from refrigerator, stir to mix, and top with toasted pumpkin seeds.

1 large sweet potato

3 large carrots

1 large yellow beet

1 large beet

Honey-Lime Vinaigrette:

½ cup extra virgin olive oil

½ lime, juiced

2 tablespoons white balsamic vinegar

1 tablespoon Dijon mustard

1 tablespoon raw or local honey

1 large clove garlic, minced

Salt and pepper to taste

Toasted pumpkin seeds for topping

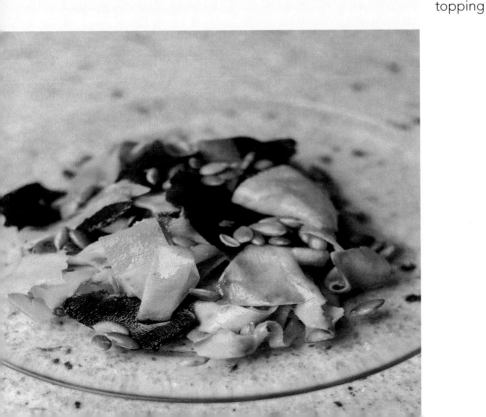

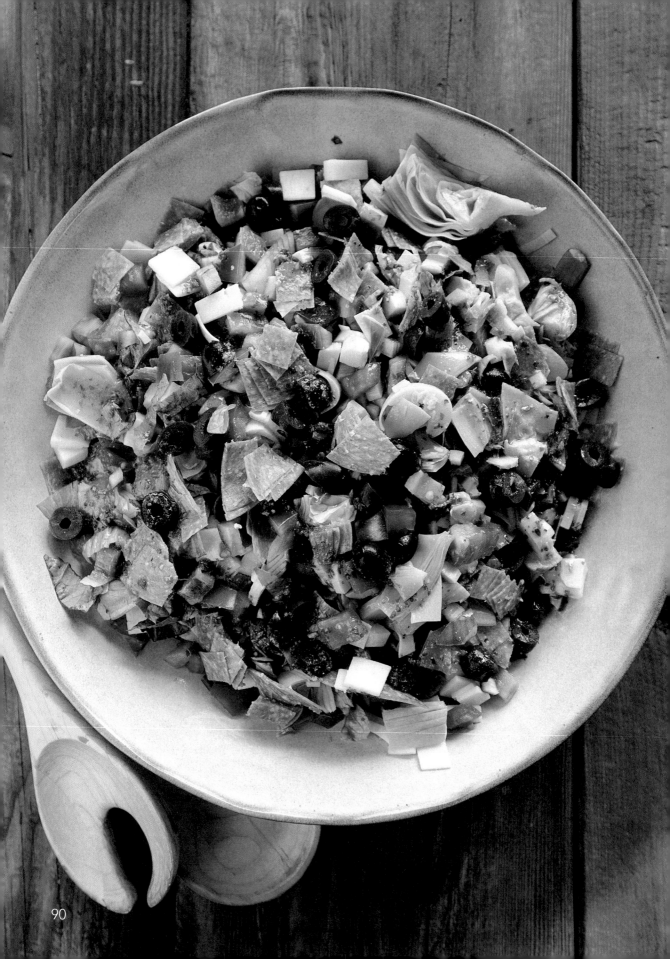

garbage chopped salad

Serves 4

Combine all salad ingredients and toss with **Herb & Red Wine Vinaigrette** below.

tip ▶ This garbage salad or "kitchen-sink" recipe was created by adding a hodgepodge of ingredients to make a creation that just works.

3 hearts romaine lettuce, diced

2 Roma tomatoes, chopped

1 green bell pepper, diced

½ red onion, chopped

½ cup pitted Kalamata olives

1 4-ounce roll Italian salami, chopped into ½-inch pieces

1 4-ounce provolone cheese, chopped into ½-inch pieces

1 can artichokes, drained and sliced

1 can hearts of palm, drained and chopped

herb & red wine vinaigrette

Mix together dressing ingredients and toss into salad mixture.

½ cup red wine vinegar

½ cup extra virgin olive oil

1 teaspoon Dijon mustard

2 garlic cloves, diced

2 tablespoons fresh basil, chopped

1 tablespoon fresh parsley, chopped

¼ teaspoon honey

Sea salt & black pepper to taste

wheat berry salad

Serve 4-6

1 cup wheat berries, rinsed and drained

3½ cups water

¼ cup balsamic vinegar

¼ cup extra virgin olive oil

Sea salt & black pepper to taste

1 tablespoon fresh chopped basil

½ cup dried cherries

¼ cup green onions, chopped

¼ cup parsley, chopped

Garnish with ¼ cup each pomegranate seeds, crumbled goat cheese and pumpkin seeds

Add wheat berries and water to small soup pot. Bring to a boil over high heat. Reduce heat to low, cover and cook for 1 hour until wheat berries are cooked and liquid is absorbed. Let cool for 10 minutes.

Add balsamic, oil, salt, black pepper, and basil to the cooled wheat berries. Stir to mix.

Add cherries, onions, parsley and stir to combine.

Chill in refrigerator overnight or serve immediately.

Top with pomegranate seeds, goat cheese, and pumpkin seeds.

 Did you know wheatgrass comes from the wheat berry?

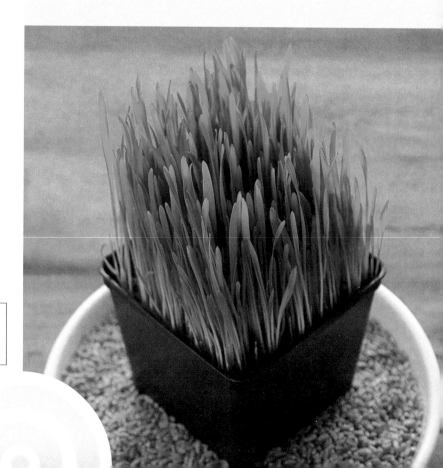

quinoa salad with pistachios & cranberries

Serves 4

Toast the quinoa in a 4-quart pot over high heat, shaking the pan occasionally, until the quinoa is light brown, starts to crackle, and smells a bit toasted, about 5 minutes.

Add the water to the toasted quinoa, cover and bring to a simmer. Cook until the quinoa is soft but still has a little bite, about 15 minutes. The water should be totally absorbed.

Transfer quinoa to a bowl and let cool slightly. Once the quinoa has cooled, add the pistachio nuts, celery, scallions, and cranberries, and toss everything together.

Dress the salad with the **Dijon Mustard Vinaigrette** below.

If not serving immediately, refrigerate the salad, but bring it to room temperature before serving.

1 cup quinoa

1½ cups water

⅓ cup pistachio nuts

2 stalks celery, sliced

3 scallions, green tops removed, sliced

¼ cup dried cranberries, coarsely chopped

 Quinoa is so versatile. You can eat it warm or cold, and it blends with many flavors. Try using it as substitute for any grain or pasta.

dijon mustard vinaigrette

Whisk together vinegar, Dijon mustard, sea salt, and black pepper in a small deep bowl. Slowly pour in the extra virgin olive oil into the bowl while whisking until dressing has emulsified.

2 tablespoons white wine vinegar

1 tablespoon Dijon mustard

¼ teaspoon sea salt

Black pepper

¼ cup extra virgin olive oil

macho salad

Serves 4

2 boneless, skinless chicken breasts, cut into cubes

1 tablespoon herbes de Provence

1 tablespoon extra virgin olive oil

2 heads romaine lettuce, chopped

½ head red cabbage, chopped

2 avocados, chopped

1 cup trail mix (dried cranberries, pistachios, almonds)

½ cup pitted dates, chopped

Season chicken with herbes de Provence and sauté in olive oil. Remove chicken from pan and set aside.

Sauté red cabbage in olive oil in the same pan you cooked the chicken, and set aside.

Mix all ingredients together in a large bowl and top with **Citrus Vinaigrette** below.

tip▶ This salad is a perfect combination of savory and sweet. It is a salad full of strong characteristics and flavors, making it "macho".

citrus vinaigrette

½ cup red wine vinegar

½ orange, juiced

⅓ cup extra virgin olive oil

½ tablespoon honey

Sea salt to taste

Combine dressing ingredients in a food processor and mix well.

kale caesar salad

Serves 4

Chop kale into small pieces and add to a large salad bowl.

In a small skillet over medium-low heat, brown breadcrumbs with 1 tablespoon extra virgin olive oil until crispy.

Drizzle **Caesar Dressing** below onto kale and massage into the salad. Your hands actually work best. The more you handle and stir the kale the softer it will be and the dressing will absorb into the leaves.

Top kale salad with bread crumbs and parmesan cheese.

tip ▶ May use hemp seeds in place of breadcrumbs but do not heat. Massaging the dressing into the kale leaves will help to break down the texture of the kale so it is easier to eat.

1 large bunch kale, spines removed, rinsed and dried

¼ cup Italian seasoned panko breadcrumbs (see tip)

¼ cup parmesan cheese, shredded

caesar dressing

In a small food processor, blend all ingredients together until mixed well.

Caesar dressing is not always made with the healthiest ingredients or can contain raw egg yolk. Using Greek yogurt, Dijon mustard and garlic is a healthy way to mimic that delicious Caesar flavor.

1 (5.3 ounce) container organic Greek yogurt

1 tablespoon extra-virgin olive oil

1 lemon, juiced

¼ cup of freshly grated parmesan cheese

2 anchovies (can use jarred)

1 clove of garlic, minced

1 teaspoon Dijon mustard

¼ teaspoon sea salt

¼ teaspoon black pepper

beet salad

Served 2-4

3 medium beets, peeled and sliced

½ cucumber, peeled and sliced

4 bibb lettuce leaves or a bunch of baby spinach

1 pound block feta cheese, thinly sliced

matt: This beet salad makes non-beet lovers think twice.

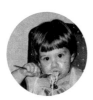

Make **Horseradish Sauce** below and put in refrigerator for 30 minutes.

Preheat oven to 350°F.

Spread beet slices on a cookie sheet in a single layer and bake for 15 minutes. Turn and cook another 15 minutes.

Place one lettuce leaf or one layer of spinach leaves on each of 4 salad plates.

Layer beets, cucumber, and feta cheese on top of spinach or lettuce, and then repeat the layers.

Top with a couple tablespoons of Horseradish Sauce below.

horseradish sauce

1 cup plain fat free Greek yogurt

2 tablespoons extra virgin olive oil

1 tablespoon prepared horseradish

Sea salt & black pepper to taste

Whisk together yogurt, horseradish, olive oil, sea salt, and black pepper together and put in refrigerator for 30 minutes.

 Greek yogurt is thicker and creamier than regular yogurt since most of the whey has been removed. Plus, it contains twice the protein of regular yogurt and less lactose as well. It also serves as a healthy substitute for mayonnaise and sour cream.

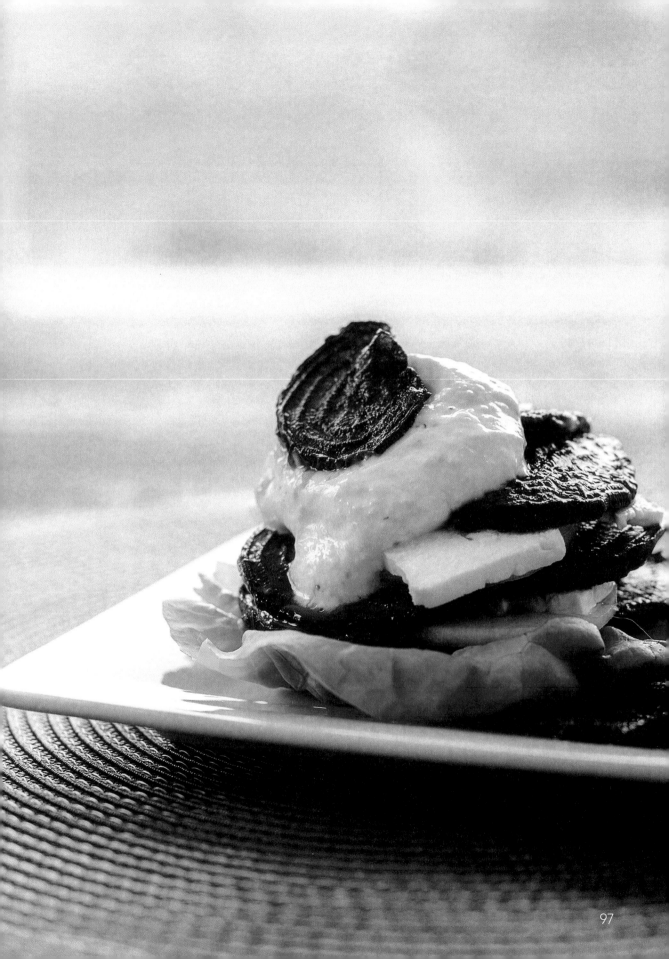

broccoli salad

Serves 4-6

1 head broccoli, chopped into small bite-sized pieces

1 cup whole almonds, toasted and coarsely chopped

¼ cup raisins

½ medium red onion, finely chopped

4 strips bacon or turkey bacon, cooked and chopped

Toss the broccoli with toasted almonds, raisins, red onion, and bacon.

Pour the **Ranch Dressing** below over the salad, and toss well.

Season with additional sea salt and black pepper to taste.

 Look for organic bacon that does not contain nitrates. Nitrates are preservatives added to bacon and cured meats to preserve color and increase shelf life.

ranch dressing/dip

¾ cup unsweetened almond milk

1 cup nonfat plain Greek yogurt

2 teaspoons onion powder

1 teaspoon garlic powder

1 tablespoon fresh dill

1 tablespoon fresh chives or diced green onions

Sea salt & black pepper to taste

Whisk all ingredients together until creamy. Refrigerate in airtight container for up to 7 days. It will thicken after refrigeration.

goddess salad

Serves 2

Heat a medium skillet over medium heat. Add in pecans and cook for 5 to 10 minutes or until toasted. Turn off heat and drizzle pecans with agave nectar. Let sit for 10 minutes.

Combine all salad ingredients and toss to mix.

Toss salad with **Dijon Mustard Vinaigrette** below and mix well.

tip▶ Serve with grilled chicken or salmon.

¼ cup pecans

1 tablespoon agave nectar or honey

2 hearts romaine lettuce, washed and chopped

½ cup hearts of palm, drained and chopped

¼ cup dried cherries

¼ cup red onion, chopped

½ cup cherry tomatoes, halved

dijon mustard vinaigrette

Whisk together vinegar, Dijon mustard, sea salt, and black pepper in a small deep bowl. Slowly pour in the extra virgin olive oil into the bowl while whisking until dressing has emulsified.

2 tablespoons white wine vinegar

1 tablespoon Dijon mustard

¼ teaspoon sea salt

Black pepper

¼ cup extra virgin olive oil

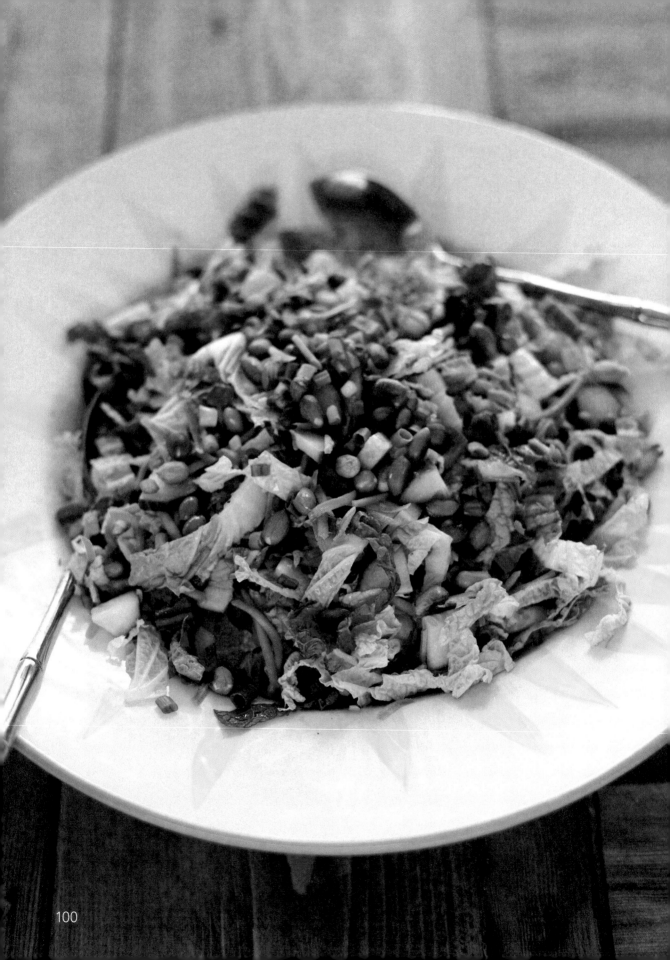

thai peanut salad

Serves 6

Prepare **Soy Awesome Dressing** below and let sit in refrigerator 10-30 minutes.

Wash and chop the cabbage, green onions, cucumber, and carrots, and place in large salad bowl.

Leave some green onions to top the salad

Use a small fry pan to warm the raw peanuts (3-5 minutes); be careful not to burn them.

Dress the salad with as much dressing as you desire. Save any unused dressing fur future use.

Top the salad with the roasted peanuts and sprinkle on the reserved green onion.

1 bunch napa cabbage

1 bunch green onions

1 cup carrots, shredded

1 cucumber, diced

½ cup pan roasted peanuts

matt: I came up with this recipe after visiting Paris of all places. I stumbled upon a food truck down by the Seine River and ordered a Thai Peanut Salad. Since I loved everything about this salad, I created this recipe in tribute.

soy awesome dressing

Whisk all ingredients together in a small mixing bowl.

Let sit for 10-30 minutes in refrigerator.

1 tablespoon rice vinegar

½ cup extra virgin olive oil

1 tablespoon toasted sesame oil

2 teaspoons Braggs Liquid Aminos or soy sauce

1 teaspoon garlic, minced

Sea salt & black pepper

 Choose organic or "Certified Non-GMO" when using soy and soy sauce products. Bragg's Liquid Aminos is a healthier non-GMO alternative to soy sauce and contains less sodium.

black bean mango salad

Serves 6

¼ cup extra virgin olive oil

¼ cup balsamic vinegar

Juice of 1 lime

2 15-ounce cans black beans, rinsed and drained (see note)

1 15-ounce can whole kernel corn, drained

1 green bell pepper, chopped

1 red pepper, chopped

½ cup green onions, chopped

2 avocados, cubed

2 mangos, peeled and chopped

Sea salt & black pepper to taste

Mix olive oil, vinegar, and lime juice in the bottom of a large mixing bowl.

Add remaining ingredients and toss to coat with dressing.

Refrigerate 1 hour before serving.

Serve as a salad or dip with organic blue corn tortilla chips.

tip▶ Can be made in advance. Leave out avocado until ready to serve.

 Rinsing and draining beans can reduce the sodium content by 40%.

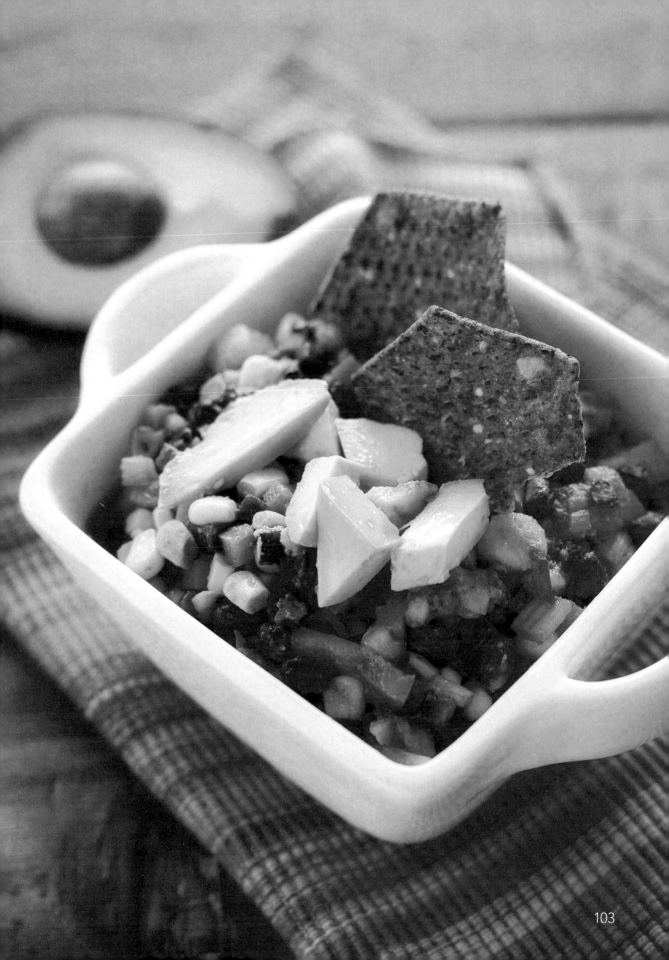

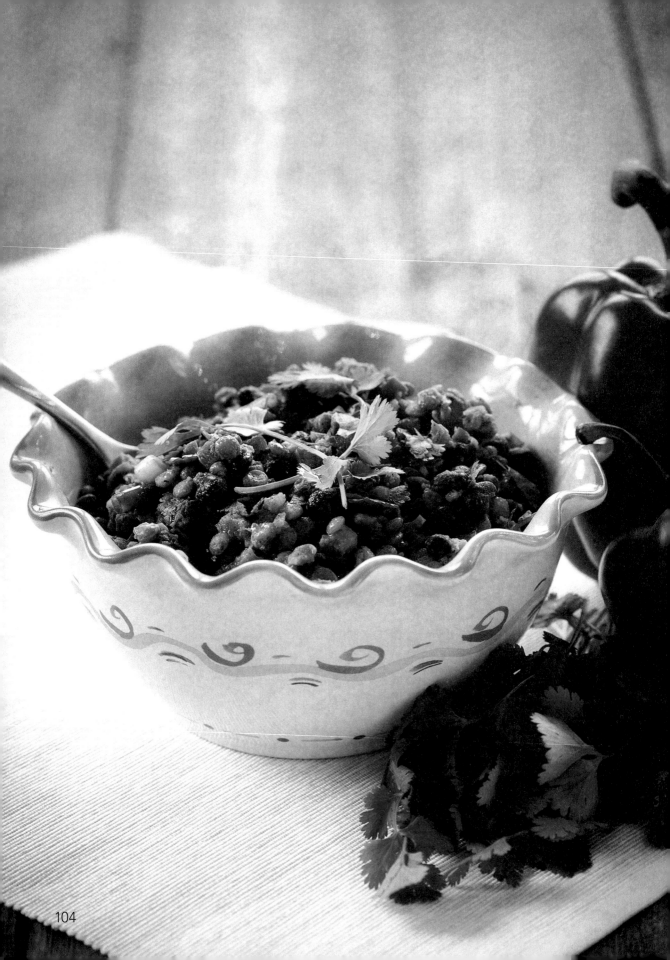

lentil & black bean salad

Serves 4-6

Put lentils into a small sauce pan with plenty of water to cover. Bring to a slow simmer and cook until lentils are tender, about 40-60 minutes for green lentils or 30-40 minutes for brown ones. Drain lentils and let cool slightly.

While lentils are cooling, rinse and drain the black beans and then dry with paper towel.

Mix chicken stock, Dijon mustard, lime juice, Worcestershire sauce, and garlic together in a small bowl.

Grind together cumin seed, chili powder, herb seasoning salt, and black pepper and add to bowl with chicken stock mixture.

Slowly drizzle olive oil into the stock mixture while whisking vigorously. Add hot sauce to taste.

When lentils are slightly cooled, add the black beans and half of the dressing and let marinate while you prep the rest of the ingredients.

Add the red pepper and green onions to lentil and bean mixture.

Stir in the rest of the dressing and add the chopped cilantro.

Salad is best if refrigerated for an hour before serving but can be served immediately.

1 cup (about ½ pound) lentils, rinsed and drained

1 can black beans, rinsed and drained

2 tablespoons chicken stock

1 teaspoon Dijon mustard

1 tablespoon fresh lime juice (can use apple cider vinegar)

1 teaspoon Worcestershire sauce

1 teaspoon garlic, finely minced

1 teaspoon cumin

½ teaspoon ancho chili powder (or any mild chili powder)

½ teaspoon of your favorite herb seasoning mix

Black pepper to taste

2 tablespoons extra virgin olive oil

Hot sauce to taste

1 cup red bell pepper, finely chopped

½ cup green onion (scallions) green part only, finely chopped

1 cup fresh cilantro, finely chopped

basil parmesan tuna salad

Serves 4 (pictured at right)

2 5-ounce cans tongol tuna in water

1 tablespoon parmesan cheese, grated

½ cup red pepper, chopped small

½ green onion, chopped

Sea salt & black pepper to taste

5 fresh basil leaves, chopped

1-2 tablespoons extra virgin olive oil

Juice of ½ lemon

Mix together and let sit in refrigerator for 1 hour before serving.

> Tongol tuna contains lower mercury levels than other tunas and is produced using responsible fishing practices. Most of all, tongol tuna has a much fresher taste than other canned tunas.

super easy tuna salad

Serves 4

2 cans tongol or wild caught tuna, drained

¼ cup dill pickles, chopped

¼ cup celery, diced

¼ cup green onions, diced

¼ cup extra virgin or avocado oil mayonnaise

Mix all ingredients in a large bowl. Serve with crackers, add to a salad, lettuce wrap, sprouted grain or coconut wrap.

tip ▶ Upgrade your processed mayonnaise to a mayonnaise made with healthier oils and cage free eggs.

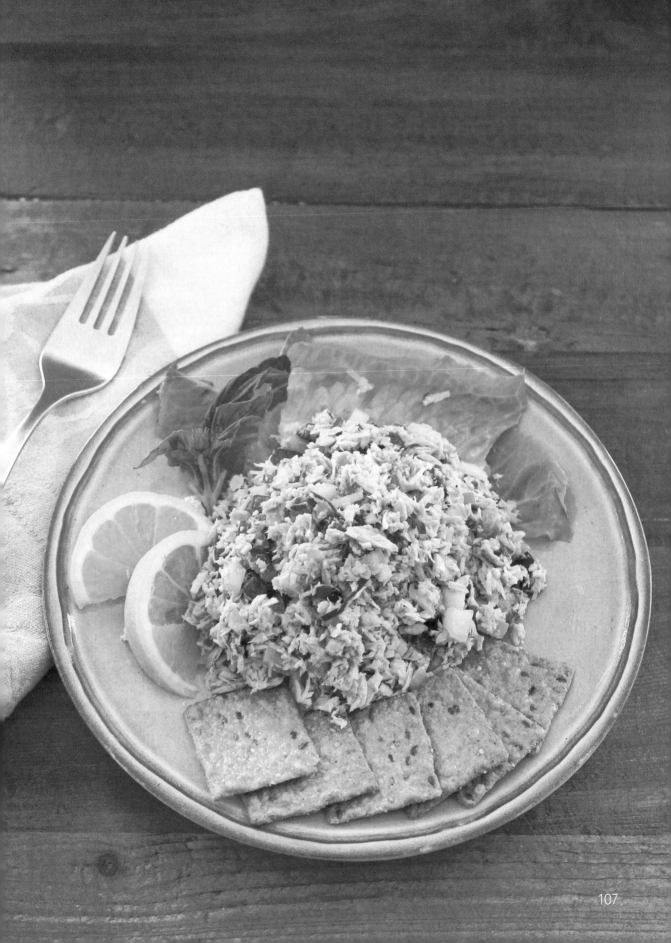

awesome chicken salad

Serves 6

For the dressing:

⅔ cup olive oil mayonnaise

Juice of ½ lemon

2 tablespoons curry powder
(more or less to taste)

Sea salt & black pepper
to taste

For the salad:

4 boneless, skinless chicken
breasts (poached in broth),
cooled and chopped

½ cup black or wild rice
(cooked and cooled)

1 cup celery, chopped

4 scallions, chopped

1 cup walnuts chopped

¾ cup dried cranberries or
cherries

Whisk together mayonnaise, lemon juice, curry powder, and salt and black pepper. Store in the refrigerator 1 hour before mixing with remaining ingredients.

Mix all ingredients in a large bowl and combine with the dressing.

tip ▶ This can be served wrapped in large lettuce leaves or collard greens.

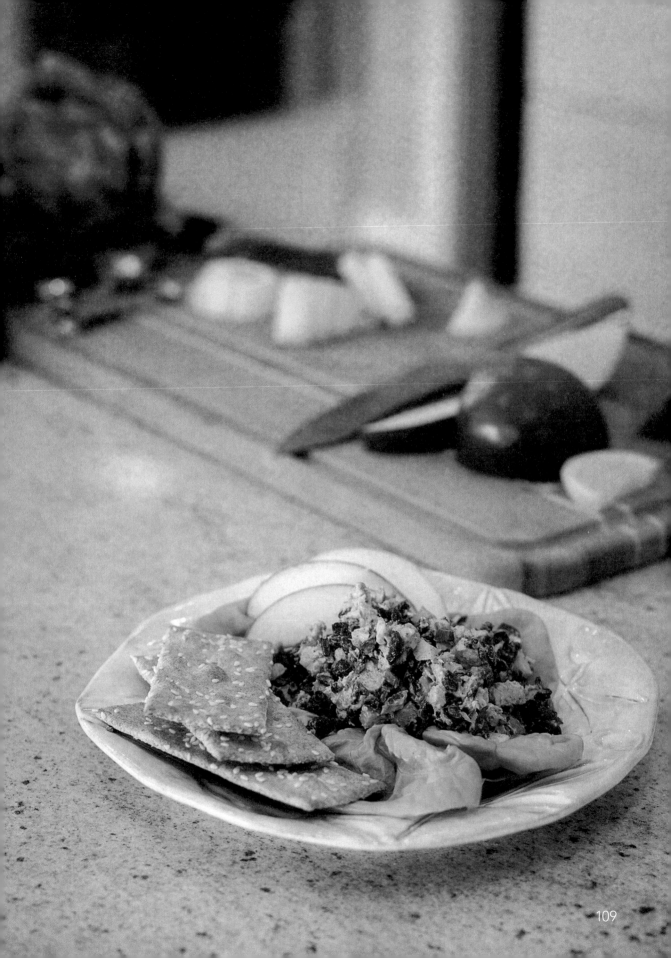

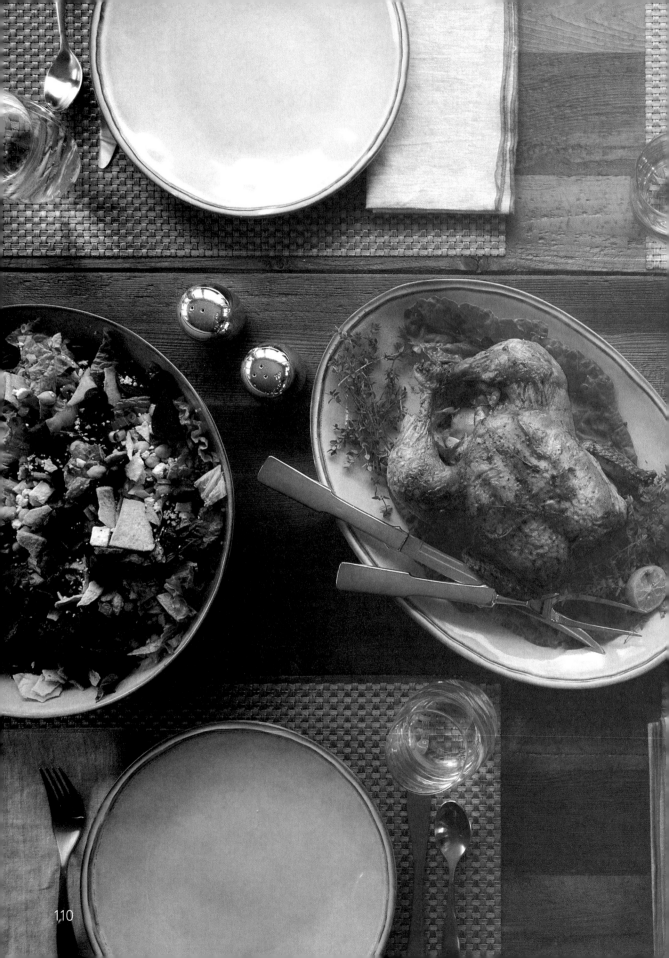

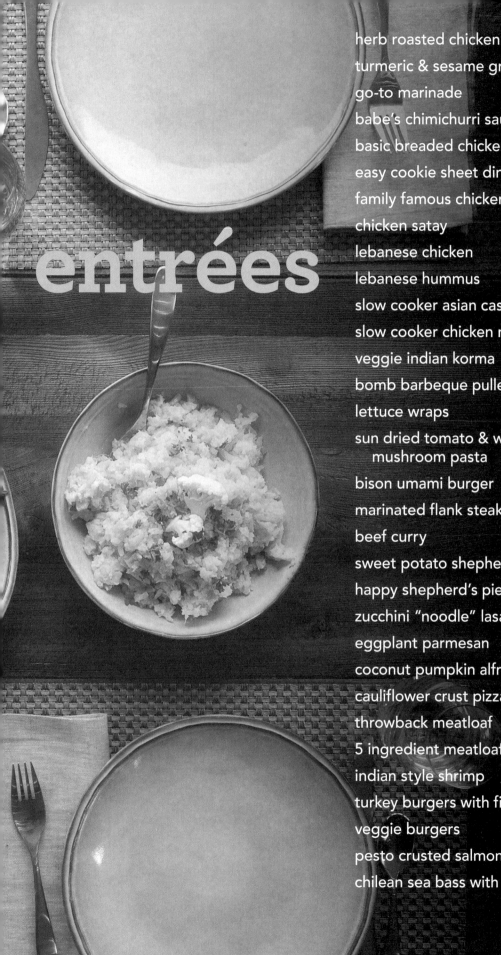

entrées

herb roasted chicken

Serves 4-6 (pictured on page 110)

1 3-4 pound whole organic chicken

4 sprigs fresh thyme or rosemary

1 lemon, quartered

1 onion, quartered

Extra virgin olive oil

Sea salt & black pepper

Preheat oven to 350°F.

Wash and dry the chicken.

Place it in a 13x9 inch roasting pan.

Gently separate the skin from the breast of the chicken to slide in one sprig of fresh thyme or rosemary on each breast.

Rub a light layer of extra virgin olive oil over entire chicken and season with salt and black pepper. Don't forget to oil and season the back side of the chicken.

Place a sprig of fresh herbs under the bird and on top.

Insert the quartered lemon and onion into the chicken cavity.

Fold the wings under the chicken, and tie the legs together.

Roast the chicken for approximately 1.5 hours until internal temperature of the thickest part of the leg reaches 160°F.

Baste occasionally with the pan drippings. Let sit for 20 minutes before carving.

Enjoy.

turmeric & sesame grilled chicken

Serves 4

Rinse chicken and pat dry.

Drizzle chicken with olive oil, and season with sea salt, black pepper, turmeric, and sesame seeds. Turn and season again on the second side.

Preheat a grill pan on medium-high.

Place the chicken on the grill pan and do not touch until the chicken is sufficiently browned. Turn chicken over and brown sufficiently on the second side.

8 boneless, skinless chicken thighs or 4 boneless, skinless chicken breasts

1 tablespoon extra virgin olive oil

Sea salt & black pepper

1 tablespoon ground turmeric

1 tablespoon sesame seeds

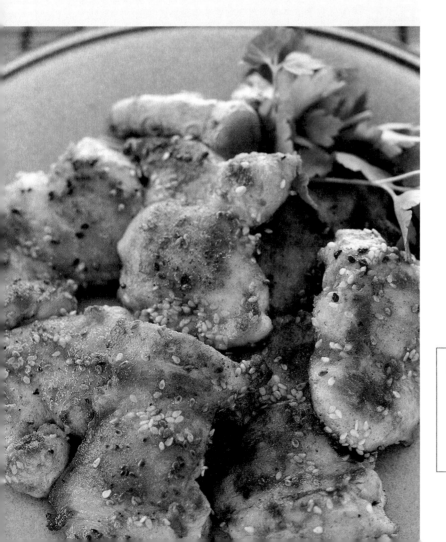

 Turmeric is one of the most powerful antioxidant-rich herbs used to help with pain, inflammation, brain health, digestion, and immune function.

113

go-to marinade

½ cup red wine vinegar

½ cup Bragg's Liquid Aminos

1 cup organic ketchup

¼ cup extra virgin olive oil

2 cloves garlic, chopped

Whisk all ingredients in a small mixing bowl.

Brush on chicken, steak, or fish, or use as a marinade for steak and chicken kabobs.

babe's chimichurri sauce

Makes 1 cup of sauce

2 heaping cups fresh parsley, chopped

2 heaping tablespoons fresh oregano

4 garlic cloves, peeled and chopped

¼ cup red wine vinegar

1 cup extra virgin olive oil

1 teaspoon salt or more to taste

Place all ingredients in a food processor and blend until slightly chunky.

Use as a sauce for steak, pasta, veggies, or seafood.

 On those nights when you need a quick chicken, steak, or fish preparation, use a bottle of salad dressing for an easy marinade. Look for salad dressings that use extra virgin olive oil or expeller pressed oils. These oils provide the most flavor and nutrition.

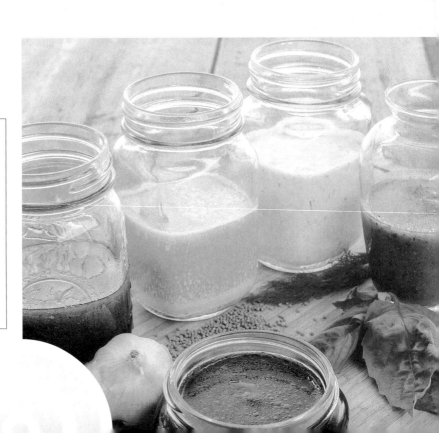

basic breaded chicken

Serves 4

Slice chicken in half lengthwise if thick. Place on a cutting board and place a sheet of saran wrap over chicken. Pound chicken with a meat mallet until flat.

Remove saran wrap and season chicken with sea salt and black pepper or favorite seasoning.

Combine egg and almond milk in a shallow bowl. Place coconut flour or breading of choice in another shallow bowl. Dip chicken in egg mixture then dry mixture, shaking off excess.

Heat a skillet with 2 tablespoons extra virgin olive oil over medium high heat. Place a single layer of the breaded chicken in the hot skillet flipping once until brown and crispy on both sides (about 4-5 minutes per side). Repeat with remaining chicken if necessary.

Place browned chicken on baking sheet and bake at 350°F for 10 minutes to ensure the chicken is cooked through and to keep warm.

1 pound boneless, skinless chicken breasts

Sea salt, black pepper, and/or favorite seasoning

1 egg

2 tablespoons unsweetened almond milk

2 cups of breading (organic unbleached all-purpose flour, coconut flour, almond flour, breadcrumbs, panko, our ground nuts)

tip ▶ To make a chicken parmesan version, simply top breaded chicken with fresh mozzarella and pasta sauce and bake at 350 degrees F for 10 minutes. Sprinkle with shredded parmesan and fresh basil.

kristen: *For nights when you simply don't know what to make for dinner—pound it, bread it, fry it, and eat it. Makes great leftovers and can be added to sandwiches or salads..*

 If using breadcrumbs, use an organic version if available.

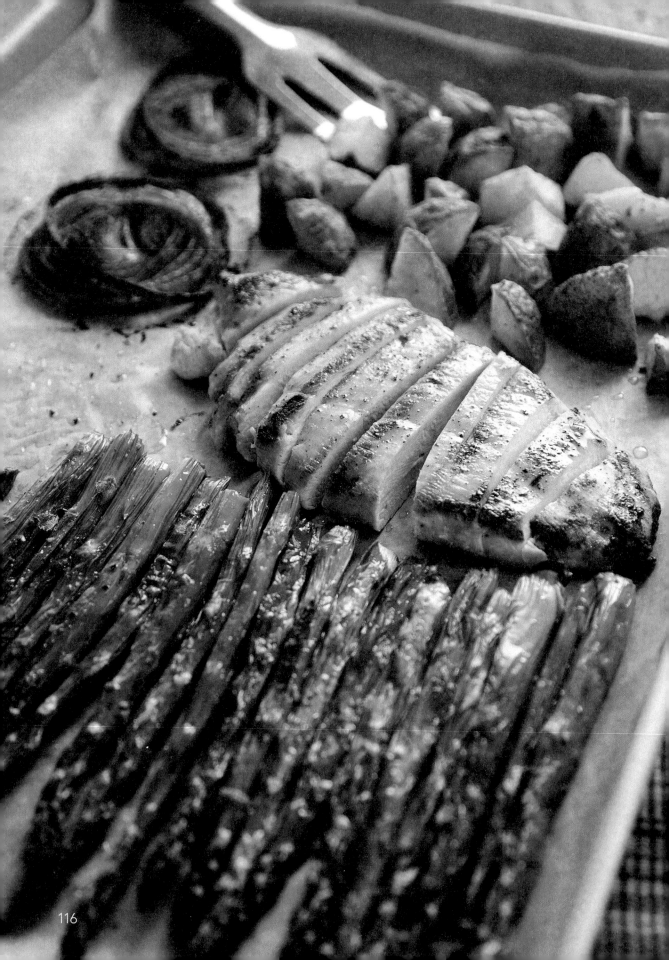

easy cookie sheet dinner

Serves 1-12

Scale to serve more.

Preheat oven to 425°F.

Lightly coat cookie sheet with olive oil.

Place potato slices on cookie sheet in a single layer; sprinkle with 1 teaspoon of extra virgin olive oil. Place cookie sheet on bottom rack in oven and roast for 10 minutes.

Remove the tray from the oven and carefully turn the potatoes.

Season the chicken breast with lemon pepper and place on the cookie sheet along with the vegetables. Roast for an additional 10 minutes.

Turn the chicken and toss the potatoes and vegetables to keep them from getting too browned.

Dinner is done when vegetables are tender and chicken is cooked through.

Season with sea salt and black pepper to taste.

1 large sweet potato or baking potato, peeled and cut into ½-inch slices or cubes

3 teaspoons extra virgin olive oil, divided

8 ounces boneless, skinless chicken breast

½ teaspoon lemon pepper

8 ounces cleaned asparagus, green beans, onions, mushrooms, broccoli, and/or any other preferred vegetables

tip ▶ This cookie sheet dinner is a great recipe for a quick weeknight meal.

family famous chicken & noodles

Serves 4

1 package boneless, skinless chicken thighs (about 6-8 pieces)

1 cup flour (as an alternate, use half almond flour and half unbleached white flour)

¼ cup parsley, chopped (reserve some for garnish)

2 eggs

2 tablespoons extra virgin olive oil

2 cups chicken broth

1 pint mushrooms, sliced

1 box whole grain pasta of choice

2 tablespoons parsley, chopped

Rinse and dry chicken. Season generously with sea salt and black pepper.

Place flour and parsley in a shallow bowl. In another shallow bowl whisk eggs.

Dip chicken into egg mixture and then in flour mixture until coated.

Heat extra virgin olive oil in a large deep fry pan over medium-high heat.

Brown chicken in olive oil 5-7 minutes per side.

Add the sliced mushrooms and chicken broth to the chicken in the pan.

Simmer over medium heat until broth thickens, about 10-12 minutes.

Meanwhile, cook pasta according to package directions.

Serve chicken and sauce over cooked pasta.

Sprinkle with fresh parsley.

kristen & matt:
We request "Chicken & Noodles" for our birthday dinner every year!

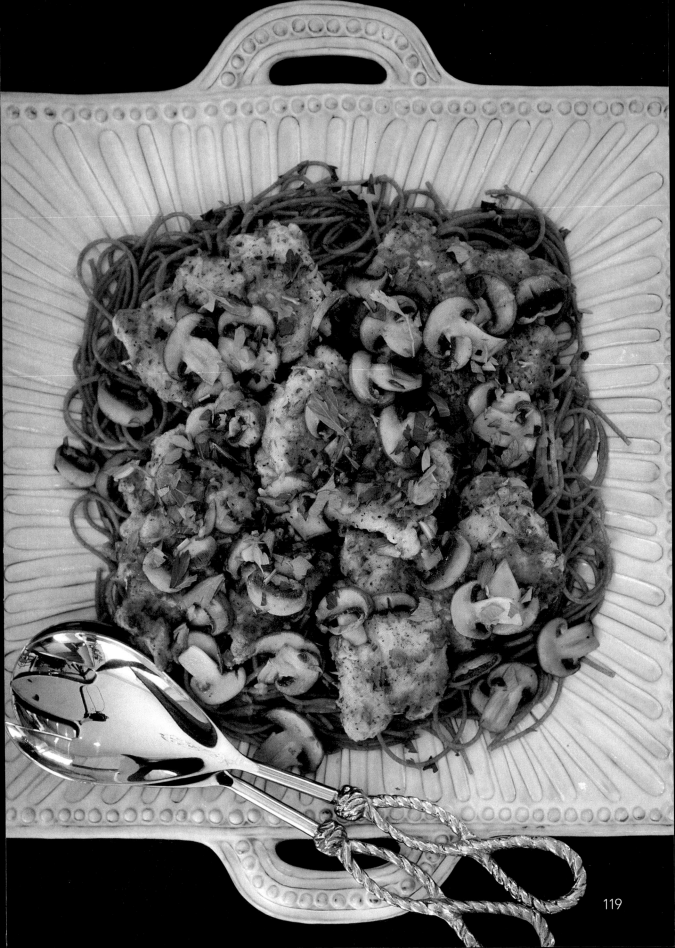

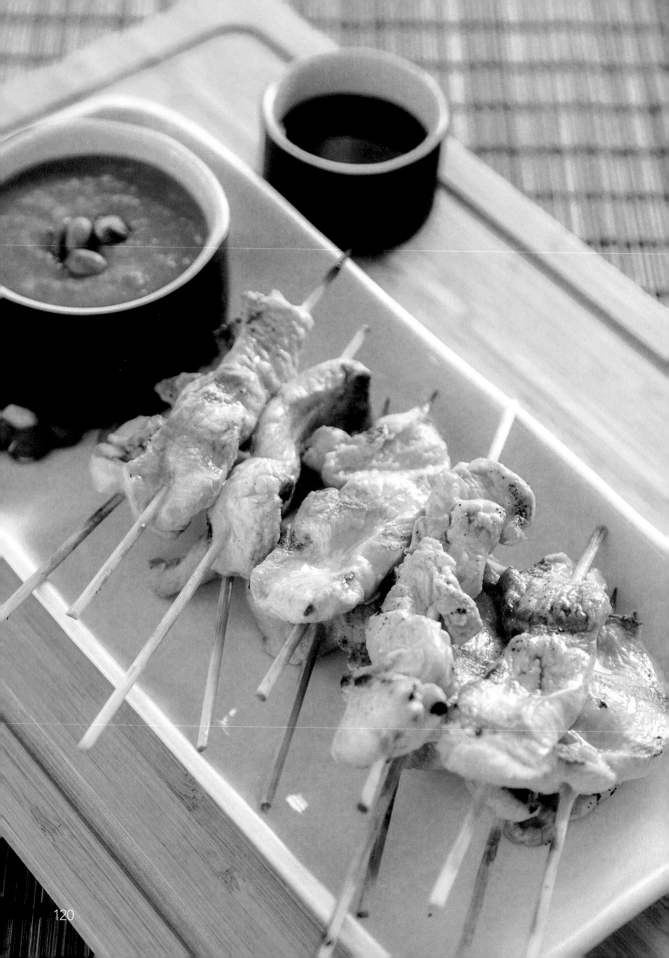

chicken satay

Serves 4

Slice the chicken thinly and arrange in a deep dish.

Mix the Bragg's, lime juice, and olive oil together well. Pour over chicken and let marinate in fridge overnight or for at least 1 hour.

Remove the chicken from the marinade and thread onto skewers.

Cook on the grill on medium-high heat until cooked through.

Meanwhile, prepare the peanut sauce by combining all ingredients. Whisk vigorously until a smooth consistency. Add more water for a thinner consistency.

Serve chicken with satay sauce.

For the chicken and marinade:

1 pound boneless, skinless chicken breasts

4 tablespoons Bragg's Liquid Aminos

1 tablespoon extra virgin olive oil

¼ cup fresh lime juice

For the peanut sauce:

¼ cup natural peanut butter

⅓ cup warm water

1 tablespoon Bragg's Liquid Aminos

1 tablespoon apple cider vinegar

1 teaspoon honey

1 teaspoon fresh ginger

tip▶ Peanut Sauce is delicious with chicken, steak, veggies, and rice.

lebanese chicken

Serves 4-6

1 package organic bone in, skin on, chicken thighs

1 tablespoon seasoning salt

1 tablespoon garlic powder

1 tablespoon paprika

1 tablespoon Lebanese Pepper Mix*

Preheat oven to 375°F.

Drizzle a little extra virgin olive oil on the bottom of a casserole dish.

Season chicken on both sides and cook chicken skin side up for 60 minutes without disturbing.

Remove from oven and use a spoon to drizzle juice from bottom of the pan over chicken.

Let cool for 10 minutes before serving. Serve with Lebanese hummus if desired.

tip ▶ For the Lebanese pepper mix, combine ¼ cup of black pepper, ¼ cup of allspice, and ¼ teaspoon ground cinnamon in a small container. Reserve leftover seasoning to use for cooking meats, and vegetables.

lebanese hummus

2 garlic cloves, peeled and pressed

1 can chickpeas, drained and rinsed

1 cup tahini

Juice of 1 lemon, may need to add more lemon to taste

1 teaspoon sea salt

⅓ cup water or more as needed for desired consistency

Place all ingredients except water into a food processor.

Blend 2-3 minutes while pouring in water until desired consistency.

Place in bowl and drizzle with extra virgin olive oil. Toasted pine nuts and paprika can also be added.

Serve with pita bread or veggie sticks.

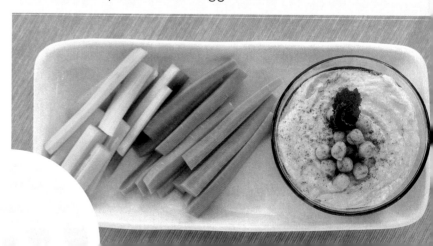

slow cooker asian cashew chicken

Serves 4-6

Combine all ingredients except cashews in a large slow cooker. Cook on high for 4 hours or on low for 8 hours or until chicken is tender.

Turn slow cooker off and let sit for 30 minutes, then pull the chicken into shreds using two forks.

Serve chicken over whole grain rice and top with cashews and a side of sautéed spinach.

 Coconut sugar is made by boiling and dehydrating the sap of the coconut palm. It contains more nutrients and is lower on the glycemic index than table sugar

¼ cup Bragg's Liquid Aminos

2 tablespoons rice vinegar

2 tablespoons organic ketchup

1 tablespoon coconut sugar

1 garlic clove, minced

1 tablespoon ginger, grated

1 package boneless, skinless chicken thighs or breasts

½ cup raw cashews

slow cooker chicken nachos

Serves 6-8

Place chicken, tomatoes with juice, chilies with juice, and taco seasoning into a slow cooker. Cook on low for 8 hours or high for 4 hours.

One half hour before serving, pull out the chicken and shred. Add chicken back into slow cooker.

Add in the beans, onions, corn and its juice if needed, and cheese. Cook for another 30 minutes on high.

Serve over tortilla chips.

2 boneless, skinless chicken breasts

1 14.5-ounce can diced tomatoes and can juice

1 4-ounce can green chilies, chopped, retain and use the juice

1 package taco seasoning (see page 83 for homemade Taco Seasoning recipe)

1 14.5-ounce can refried beans

¾ cup onion, chopped

1 14.5-ounce can sweet corn, and juice if needed

5 ounces shredded cheddar cheese

Garnish with sliced avocado or guacamole (see Guaca-Money recipe page 56) and serve with 1 bag tortilla chips

Curry Sauce:

2 tablespoons organic grass fed ghee

1 teaspoon cumin seeds

1 large onion, chopped

4 cloves garlic, minced

2 tablespoons chopped ginger

1 large tomato, chopped

1 teaspoon sea salt

1 teaspoon ground coriander

1 teaspoon paprika

1 teaspoon turmeric

1 teaspoon garam masala

½ teaspoon chili powder

¼ teaspoon ground cardamom

½ cup unsalted cashews

1 ½ cups water

Vegetables:

1 tablespoon olive oil

1 small head cauliflower, chopped into small florets

1 cup fresh green beans, chopped

4 large carrots, sliced thin

1 red bell pepper, seeds removed and chopped

To Finish:

½ cup golden raisins

½ cup unsalted cashews

1 can organic original coconut milk, use hardened cream

Cilantro chopped

veggie indian korma

Serves 4

To make curry sauce, heat ghee in a skillet over medium heat. Add cumin seeds until lightly browned, about 2 minutes, then add in onions, cooking until tender and fragrant. Add garlic, ginger, tomato, and spices. Stir to mix and then add cashews. Cook for 2-3 minutes more and let cool.

Pour mixture into a food processor or blender and puree until smooth. Add finished curry sauce to a crockpot over low heat.

To prepare vegetables, heat 1 tablespoon olive oil in large skillet. Add vegetables and saute' over medium high heat for 2-3 minutes. Cover and let steam till tender, about 5 minutes. Add to crockpot with curry sauce and cook on low for 1-2 hours.

Meanwhile, in a medium skillet, heat 1 tablespoon of ghee. Add the golden raisins, and cashews. Saute' until lightly toasted, about 2-3 minutes. Add to curry vegetable sauce along with coconut cream right before serving. Season with salt and pepper to taste.

Sprinkle on fresh chopped cilantro and serve.

bomb barbeque pulled chicken

Serves 4

Place all ingredients in slow cooker and cook on low for 6-8 hours until meat is very tender.

Pull meat apart with a fork. Top with a sprinkle of smoked paprika.

kristen: *I first served this recipe at a house party for over 50 guests! It was a huge success and I will forever remember this day. When a small town girl makes a bomb barbeque sauce, it only seems right that it should be published.*

1 package boneless, skinless chicken thighs or breasts

1 cup organic ketchup

1 tablespoon brown sugar

1 tablespoon molasses

1 tablespoon red wine vinegar

¼ teaspoon cayenne pepper

½ tablespoon garlic powder

½ tablespoon dry mustard

½ tablespoon chili powder

½ teaspoon black pepper

½ teaspoon ground allspice

½ teaspoon ground cinnamon

1 onion, chopped

Sea salt to taste

Smoked paprika

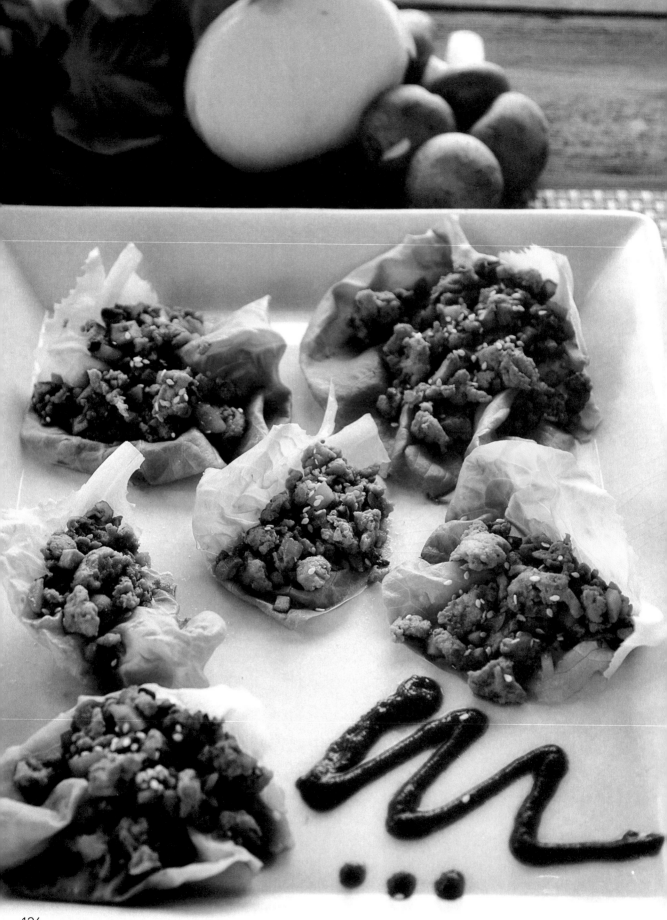

126

lettuce wraps

Serves 4

Brown the ground chicken with 1 tablespoon olive oil in a large sauté pan over medium-high heat.

Add remaining 1 tablespoon olive oil to another medium pan and sauté the yellow onions, mushrooms, and water chestnuts until the mushrooms become tender.

Once the chicken is cooked thoroughly, add in the cooked mushrooms, onions, and water chestnuts mixture. Add the sesame teriyaki sauce and heat 2-3 minutes until combined

Place individual lettuce leaves on a serving plate. Spoon a generous amount of the meat mixture in each lettuce leaf. Sprinkle with diced green onion and toasted sesame.

Garnish the plate with sriracha or hot sauce for added heat (optional). Goes well with brown rice on the side.

matt: *Lettuce wraps are very popular, but many people don't make them at home. I came up with this recipe by trying a bunch of lettuce wraps and deciding what flavors and textures I preferred. These are really, really good!*

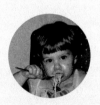

1 pound ground organic chicken

2 tablespoons extra virgin olive oil

¼ cup yellow onion, diced

1 package sliced mushrooms washed and diced

¼ cup water chestnuts, diced

2 tablespoons sesame teriyaki sauce

1 teaspoon toasted sesame seeds

½ cup green onion, sliced

1 bunch Boston lettuce, washed and separated

Garnish with sriracha or your favorite hot sauce

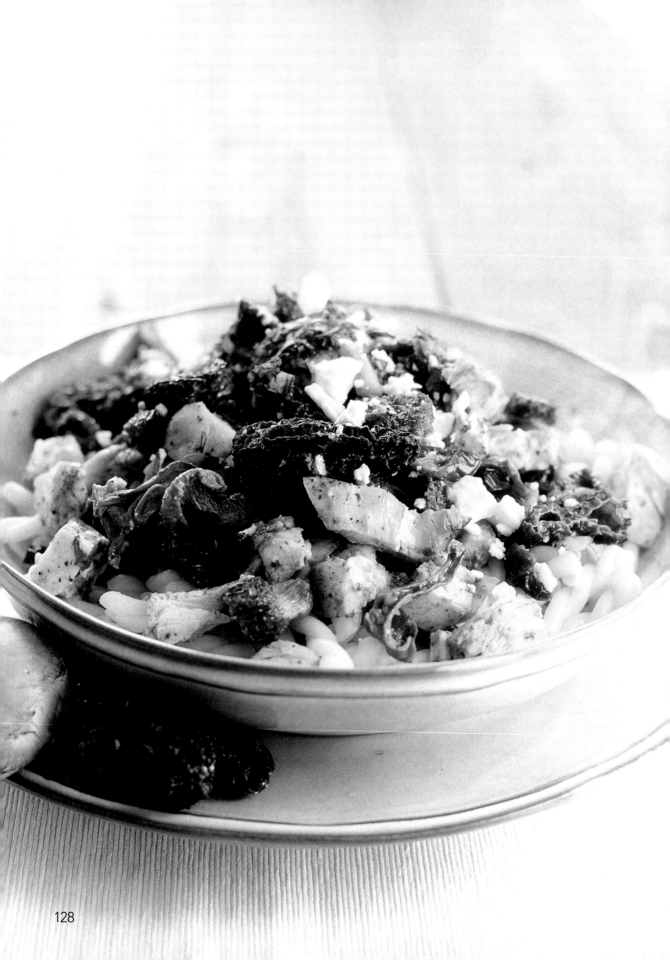

sun dried tomato & wild mushroom pasta

Serves 4-6

In small food processor place all Pesto Sauce ingredients and pulse until combined. Set aside.

Pound chicken breast to ¾-inch thickness. Lightly season chicken with sea salt and black pepper, and grill. Once grilled, slice into strips and set aside.

In a medium sauce pan boil chicken broth and Marsala wine for about 5 minutes to reduce. Once reduced, add dried mushrooms and simmer for 1-2 minutes longer. Turn off heat and let steep for 10-15 minutes. Remove the mushrooms from the broth, reserving broth.

Pour 1 cup of boiled water over the sun dried tomatoes and let soak for 2 minutes. Remove the sun dried tomatoes from the water and discard water.

Cook the pasta in boiling, salted water until al dente.

Cut the larger reconstituted mushrooms into quarters and thinly slice the sun dried tomatoes.

Heat 1 tablespoon olive oil in a large, deep sided sauté pan. Add garlic and sliced fresh mushrooms until the mushrooms have lost all of their water.

Add the dried mushrooms, chicken, and sun dried tomatoes. Season with sea salt and black pepper.

Add ½ the pesto mixture and the cooked pasta along with half of the reserved mushroom broth. Simmer until the broth evaporates slightly.

Add the remaining pesto and top with crumbled feta or goat cheese.

tip ▶ The extra pesto sauce can be stored in the refrigerator for 2 weeks.

For the pesto sauce:

2 tablespoons extra virgin olive oil

½ cup fresh basil, chopped

½ teaspoon black pepper

½ teaspoon sea salt

½ teaspoon fresh oregano

½ teaspoon fresh thyme

¼ teaspoon red pepper flakes

2 boneless, skinless chicken breasts

2 cups chicken broth

1 tablespoon Marsala wine

1 cup dried wild mushrooms (morals and northern wild)

10-12 sun dried tomatoes, dried no oil

2 cups whole wheat gemelli pasta

2 tablespoons extra virgin olive oil

1 clove garlic, chopped

1½ cups fresh mushrooms, thinly sliced

2-3 tablespoons feta cheese

bison umami burger

Serves 4

For the burgers:

1 pound ground bison

½ onion, chopped

1 tablespoon Worcestershire sauce

½ teaspoon sea salt

¼ teaspoon black pepper or 1 teaspoon steak seasoning

For the umami tapenade:

3-4 portabella mushrooms (2 cups), cut into finely diced pieces

1 tablespoon black truffle oil

Sea salt & black pepper

Additional ingredients/ toppings:

Fresh basil

Buffalo mozzarella, sliced

Tomato, sliced

Extra virgin olive oil mayonnaise

Hamburger buns

To make tapenade, heat a skillet over medium-high heat and add in mushrooms. Cover and let cook until tender, about 10 minutes. Remove pan from heat and drizzle with truffle oil. Stir to mix and reserve for later.

Preheat grill to medium-high heat.

Combine burger ingredients in a large bowl and use hands to mix. Form into 3-4 patties (depending on desired size).

Drizzle burgers with a little extra virgin olive oil to prevent from sticking and place on grill. Cook for 3-4 minutes then flip.

After 1 minute on second side, top burgers with a piece of basil and mozzarella. Continue to cook until cheese is melted, about 2 minutes. Remove from grill and let sit.

To assemble burgers, add umami tapenade to bottom of bun, and top with bison burger, tomato and a little mayo. Enjoy!

 Umami is a Japanese word that describes a meaty or savory taste. Tomatoes and mushrooms are high in free form glutamate which provides a natural umami flavor. Black truffles are a rare and extravagant mushroom with an intense meaty flavor.

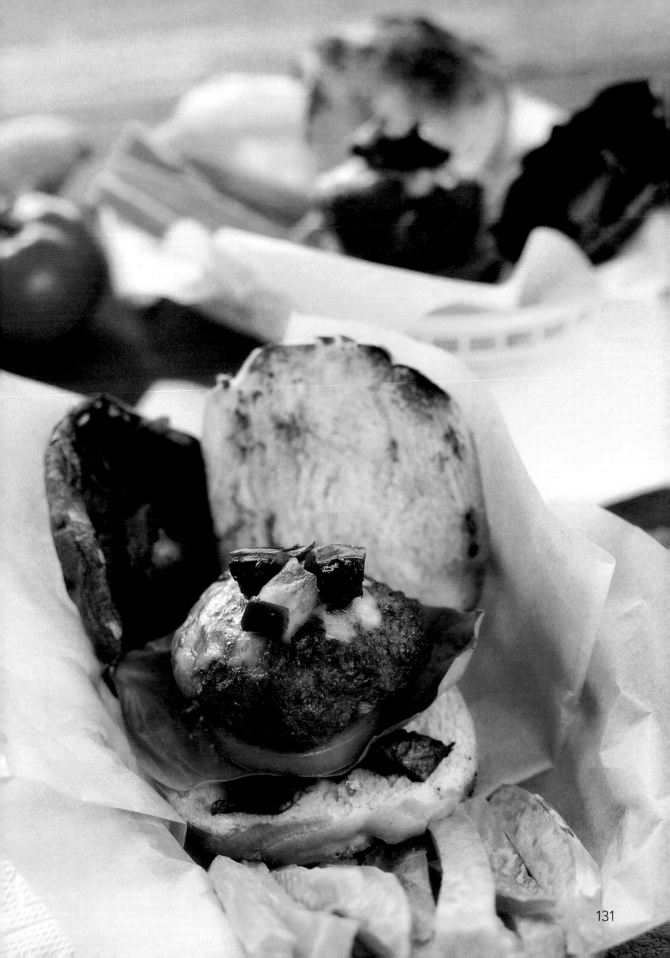

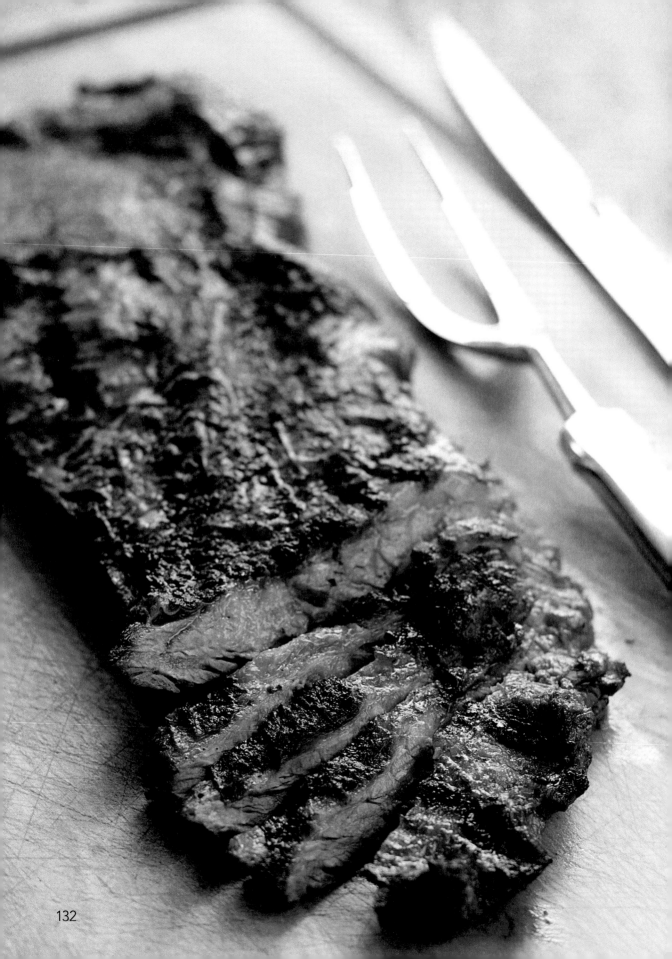

marinated flank steak

Serves 4

Mix marinade ingredients together in a large resealable plastic bag and add flank steak.

Let sit in the refrigerator overnight or for at least 4 hours.

Remove steak from refrigerator at least 20-30 minutes before grilling. To grill, remove steak from marinade and discard the marinade. Grill 5 minutes per side for medium rare.

Let steak rest at least 15 minutes before carving. To serve, cut steak diagonally across the grain into thin slices.

1.5 to 2 pound flank steak

Marinade:

½ cup extra virgin olive oil

⅓ cup Bragg's Liquid Aminos

¼ cup red wine vinegar

½ lemon, juiced

1 tablespoon Worcestershire sauce

1 teaspoon dry mustard

1 clove garlic, minced

¼ teaspoon black pepper

matt: This marinated flank steak has been the center of many special occasions at our house.

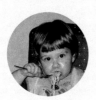

1-2 cups basmati rice

For the tzatziki sauce:

1 large English cucumber,
shredded with cheese grater

5 mint leaves, chopped

2 cups Greek yogurt

1 large clove garlic, minced

½ cup golden raisins

For the curry sauce:

1 tablespoon ground cumin

1 teaspoon ground
cinnamon

¼ teaspoon ground cloves

2 teaspoons black pepper

1 teaspoon ground turmeric

2 teaspoons paprika

¼ teaspoon cayenne

4-6 garlic cloves, chopped

1 teaspoon ginger root,
peeled and chopped

½ cup apple cider vinegar

2 tablespoons fresh parsley,
chopped

For the meat:

2 tablespoons extra virgin
olive oil

½ large red onion, sliced

1 serrano pepper, sliced
down the center, seeds
removed

2 pounds beef sirloin, cut
into ½-inch cubes

1 teaspoon sea salt

beef curry

Serves 4-6

Cook basmati rice according to package directions.

For tzatziki sauce:

Combine all ingredients in a small bowl and refrigerate
for 20-30 minutes.

To prepare the curry sauce:

Combine the cumin, cinnamon, cloves, black pepper,
turmeric, paprika, and cayenne in a mini food processor.
Add the garlic, ginger, and apple cider vinegar, and mix
until combined. Set aside.

To assemble:

Cook onions in Dutch oven over medium heat until
tender. Add the sliced serrano peppers and sauté for an
additional 12 minutes. Keep stirring, don't let the onions
burn.

Add the curry sauce to the onion and peppers, and
continue stirring for about 2 minutes or until the mixture
thickens and the moisture has evaporated. Add 1 cup
warm water to the food processor and mix to take up
the remaining spices.

Add the cubed meet to the onion and pepper mixture.
Stir occasionally for 5 minutes while the meat cooks and
gathers the curry sauce. Add sea salt to taste.

Add the water from the processor to the beef mixture.
Bring to a boil, then lower the heat to simmer for 30
minutes. Add the chopped parsley and remove from heat.

Serve over basmati rice and top with the tzatziki sauce.

matt: *This is a great recipe to start with if you
have never cooked with curry. My wife Holly and
I stumbled upon an Indian restaurant on a side
street in Old Town Nice, France. That visit inspired
this recipe.*

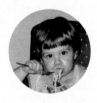

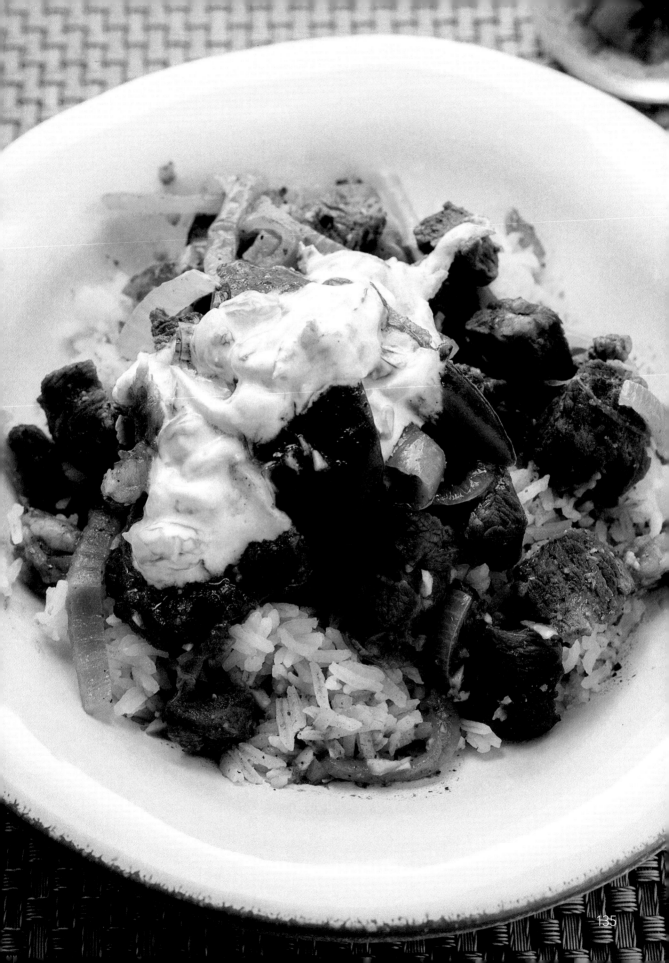

sweet potato shepherd's pie

Serves 6

3 large sweet potatoes

1 tablespoon extra virgin olive oil

1 large onion, diced

1 green bell pepper, diced

3 cloves garlic, minced

1 pound ground bison

1 package taco seasoning (or use Taco Seasoning recipe on page 83)

1 14.5 ounce can diced tomatoes

2 cups shredded cheddar cheese, divided

½ cup original coconut milk

Preheat oven to 375°F.

Place sweet potatoes on a baking sheet lined with aluminum foil and bake for 90 minutes or until sweet potatoes are tender. Remove sweet potatoes and set aside to cool. Turn the oven up to 400°F.

Meanwhile, in a large skillet heat 1 tablespoon extra virgin olive oil over medium heat. Add the onion, pepper, and garlic. Season with sea salt and black pepper, and cook until tender, about 5-7 minutes. Remove vegetables to a plate and set aside.

Add bison to skillet and sprinkle with taco seasoning. Heat until cooked through and browned. Add in the cooked vegetables and canned tomatoes. Cook for 5 minutes or until mixture comes to a low boil.

Peel the cooled sweet potatoes and add to a large bowl. Blend slightly with a hand-held mixer, and then add the coconut milk and continue to blend until the potato mixture is creamy. Stir in 1 cup of cheese.

Spray a large casserole dish with cooking spray. Spread bison mixture evenly on the bottom of casserole dish and sprinkle with the remaining cheese. Spoon the sweet potato mixture evenly over the top. Bake for 10 minutes and turn on low broil cooking for 10 minutes more or until slightly browned on top.

 Traditional Shepherd's Pie is usually made with mashed white potatoes. Using sweet potatoes instead is a tasty way to add more vitamin A, vitamin C, calcium, and iron.

tip ▶ Reach for this when you simply need a comfort food fix.

happy shepherd's pie

Serves 4

Preheat oven to 400°F.

Drizzle potato skins with olive oil, salt and pepper. Bake potatoes on a parchment lined baking sheet for 1 hour or until soft. Set aside to cool slightly.

Meanwhile, heat olive oil in a large skillet. Add peppers, onions, carrots and cook on medium high heat for about 10 minutes. Add mushrooms to the skillet, and continue to cook until vegetables are tender, about 5-10 minutes. Add in herbs de provence and season to taste with salt and pepper.

Remove vegetable mixture from skillet and set aside. Using the same skillet, add 1 tablespoon of extra virgin olive oil. Brown turkey until cooked through. Season with salt and pepper to taste. Add vegetable mixture to turkey in skillet.

Once potatoes are cooled, slice in half. Scoop the inside into a large mixing bowl. (May reserve skins for future use). Add coconut cream and green onions to potatoes and mix with a hand-held mixer until soft and creamy. Salt to taste.

Coat a large casserole dish with avocado oil spray. Spread the turkey/vegetable mixture on the bottom of dish. Top with cheese and spread mashed potatoes evenly over the top.

Bake for 15 minutes. Broil on high for 5-10 minutes until potatoes are browned. Let cool for 5 minutes before serving.

4 large russet potatoes

1 green bell pepper, chopped

1 red bell pepper, chopped

1 onion, chopped

3 large carrots, chopped

1 tablespoon herbs de provence

1 pint mushrooms, chopped

1 pound organic ground turkey

½ cup coconut cream (reserve the hardened cream from a can of original, unsweetened coconut milk)

¼ cup green onions, chopped

½ cup pepper jack cheese, shredded

tip ▶ Did you know that potatoes boost serotonin and make you feel happy?

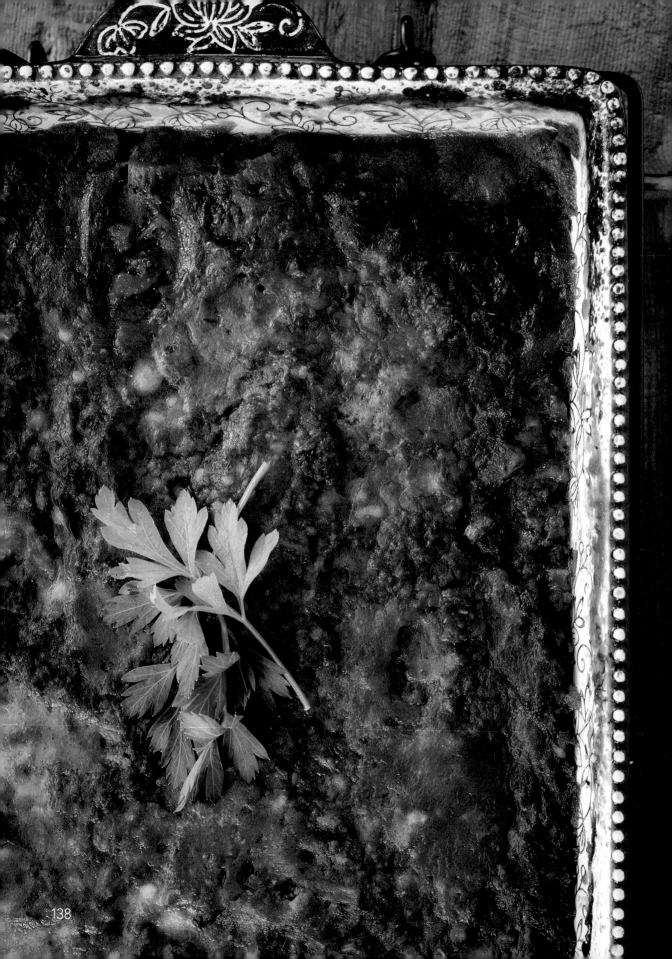

zucchini "noodle" lasagna

Serves 8-10

Brown meat in the olive oil. Add onion, celery, and garlic, and sauté for 5 minutes until translucent. Stir in tomatoes, broth, tomato paste, hot sauce, black pepper, thyme, basil, sea salt, and bay leaves. Bring to a boil; reduce heat, and simmer uncovered for 35 minutes, stirring occasionally. Stir in parsley and cook for another 2 minutes. Discard bay leaves and set sauce aside.

Place oven rack on the bottom. Preheat oven to 450°F.

Coat a large cookie sheet with extra virgin olive oil. To make zucchini "noodles," wash zucchini and cut ends off; cut lengthwise into ½-inch thick slices. Arrange zucchini slices on cookie sheet; sprinkle with ½ tablespoon olive oil and sprinkle with black pepper. Roast in oven for 10 minutes. Turn slices over and roast for an additional 5-10 minutes or until tender and nicely browned. Remove pan from oven and set aside.

Reduce oven temperature to 350°F.

Combine cottage cheese, ½ cup parmesan cheese, and egg white in a small bowl and set aside.

Brush a 9x13 inch glass baking dish with olive oil. Add a thin layer of sauce to cover the bottom. Layer half of the zucchini slices, half of the cottage cheese mixture, and half the shredded mozzarella. Spread half of the sauce over the layers, and then repeat starting with zucchini. Sprinkle 2 tablespoons parmesan cheese on top.

Bake uncovered for 20 minutes or until slightly browned and bubbly. Remove the dish from the oven and let it rest for 15 minutes before serving.

tip ▶ This can be frozen before baking for up to 1 month. Hard textured vegetables are great substitutes for white lasagna noodles.

For the sauce:

1 tablespoon extra virgin olive oil

2 pounds ground bison, turkey, or turkey Italian sausage

2 cups onions, chopped

1 cup celery, chopped

4 large cloves garlic, minced

2 14.5-ounce cans Italian stewed tomatoes

1 14.5-ounce can beef or chicken broth

1 6-ounce can tomato paste

Hot sauce to taste

½ teaspoon black pepper

½ teaspoon dried thyme

1 teaspoon dried sweet basil

⅛ teaspoon sea salt

2 bay leaves

¼ cup fresh Italian flat leaf parsley, chopped

For the lasagna:

1 pound (3 medium) zucchini

½ teaspoon black pepper

1 tablespoon extra virgin olive oil

1 cup low-fat cottage cheese or ricotta cheese

1 egg white, slightly beaten

½ cup plus 2 tablespoons parmesan cheese, grated

1 cup (4 ounces) part-skim mozzarella cheese, shredded

eggplant parmesan

Serves 4

1 medium eggplant, peeled and cut into 1-inch thick round slices

2 eggs, beaten slightly in a flat bowl

½ cup breadcrumbs

1 teaspoon sea salt

1 teaspoon black pepper

1 teaspoon garlic powder

1 teaspoon onion powder

½ cup parmesan cheese

2 cups tomato sauce or prepared spaghetti sauce (or use Lasagna Sauce on page 139)

Pre-heat oven to 350°F

Combine all dry ingredients (except for cheese) and spread evenly on a plate.

Dredge the eggplant in the egg and then the breadcrumb mixture.

Place the breaded eggplant in a single layer on a slightly oiled cookie sheet. Bake for 5 minutes on each side.

Broil the eggplant until it turns crispy and golden brown then turn and brown the other side. Once the eggplant is lightly browned on the second side, sprinkle with parmesan cheese and continue to broil until cheese is melted.

Pour heated tomato sauce over eggplant and serve.

 When you see recipes calling for breadcrumbs, flour, sauces, spices, etc., follow the Food Target and select the highest quality possible. Don't make this with the typical store-bought trans fat breadcrumbs. Make or buy real organic breadcrumbs.

coconut pumpkin alfredo sauce

Serves 4

1 14-ounce can coconut milk

1 14-ounce can pureéd pumpkin

Sea salt & black pepper to taste

1 teaspoon garlic powder

1 teaspoon onion powder

Garnish with chopped fresh chives

Combine all ingredients in a small saucepan and bring to a low simmer. Add to your favorite pasta, gnocchi, tortellini, or ravioli. Sprinkle with fresh chives.

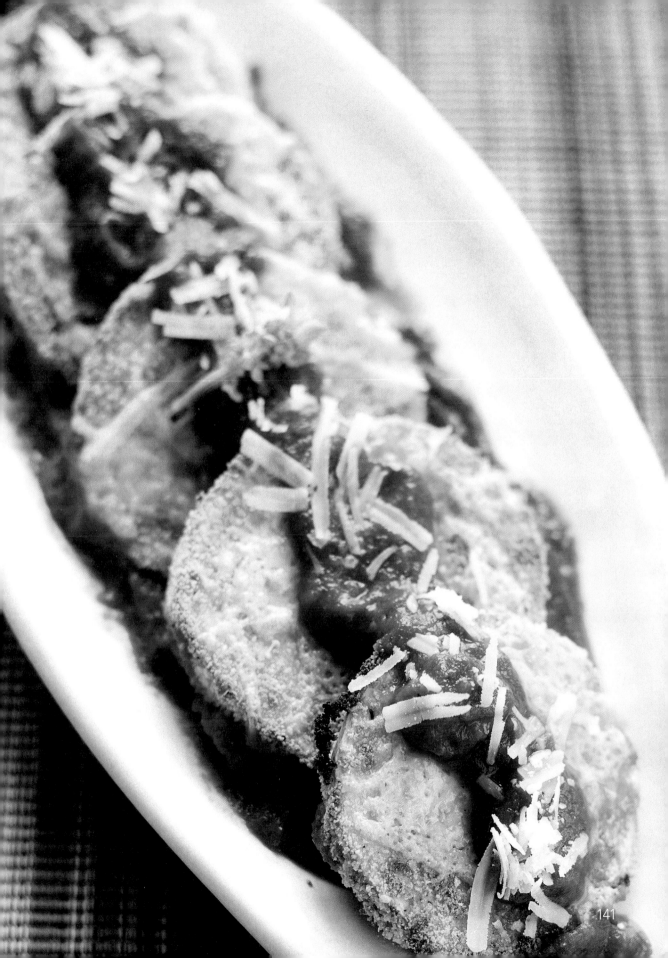

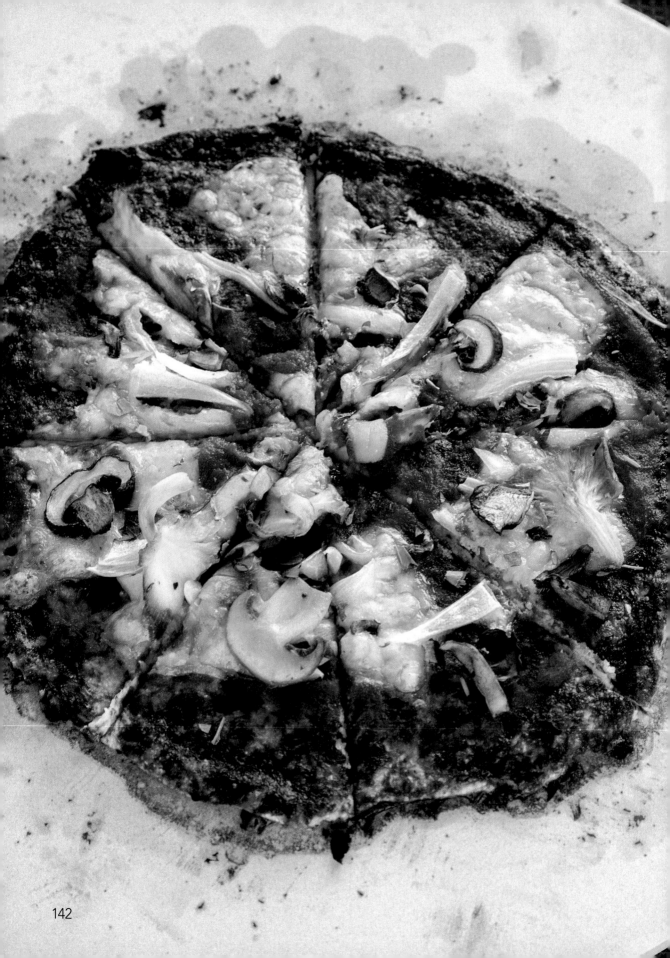

cauliflower crust pizza

Serves 4

To prepare the crust:

Preheat the oven to 450°F.

Spray a cookie sheet or pizza stone with nonstick extra virgin olive oil spray (or use a nonstick surface).

Shred the cauliflower into small crumbles. You can use a food processor if you wish, but be careful not to over process. You want dry crumples, not a purée. Pat dry if needed.

In a medium bowl, mix cauliflower crumbles with the remaining crust ingredients. Pat the "crust" into a 9-12 inch round on the prepared pan. Bake for 15 minutes (or until golden).

Remove the crust from the oven and turn the heat up to broil. If crust is still watery after 15 minutes, broil on high to get moisture out. Don't let it burn!

To assemble:

Spread the sauce on top of the baked crust, leaving a ½-inch border around the edge.

Sprinkle the mozzarella cheese on top of the sauce. Top with the sliced mushrooms and onions. Broil the pizza 3 to 4 minutes, or until the toppings are hot and the cheese is melted and bubbly.

Cut into 6 slices and serve immediately.

Crust:

1½ cups cauliflower, finely chopped (about ½ large head)

1 large egg

1 cup parmesan cheese, finely shredded

1 teaspoon dried oregano

½ teaspoon dried minced garlic (or fresh garlic)

½ teaspoon onion powder

½ teaspoon sea salt

Toppings:

½ cup pizza sauce or Lasagna Sauce (see recipe on page 139)

¼ cup mushrooms of choice, thinly sliced

¼ cup yellow onions, thinly sliced

½ cup block mozzarella, crumbled

throwback meatloaf

Serves 4-6

1½ pounds ground bison or turkey

1 10-ounce package frozen chopped spinach, thawed and drained

2 egg whites

1½ teaspoons Italian seasoning

1 cup rolled oats

½ cup onions, chopped

½ cup carrots, shredded

1 small apple, shredded

⅓ cup almond or coconut milk

½ teaspoon sea salt

¼ teaspoon black pepper

¼ cup tomato salsa or organic ketchup

Preheat oven to 350°F. Combine all ingredients in a large bowl and mix thoroughly.

Press into a 9 inch loaf pan.

Bake for 45-50 minutes or until internal temperature reaches 160°F. Spread ¼ cup tomato salsa or organic ketchup on meatloaf during last 15 minutes of baking.

Let stand 5 minutes before slicing.

tip ▶ For burgers, form into patties and broil, bake, or grill as desired.

5 ingredient meatloaf

Serves 4

1 pound ground turkey or bison

2 eggs

1 12-ounce can organic cream of mushroom soup

1 cup rolled oats

¾ cup onions, chopped

Sea salt & black pepper to taste

Preheat oven to 350°F.

Combine all ingredients and mix gently by hand.

Press into loaf pan and bake for 50 minutes, until cooked through.

indian style shrimp

Serves 2-3

Cook the basmati rice according to package directions. Five minutes before the rice is done, add the diced Roma tomatoes and chopped cilantro. Cover and finish cooking the rice.

Season the shrimp with curry, sea salt, black pepper, and cayenne pepper. Heat olive oil over medium heat in a shallow fry pan. Add the seasoned shrimp to the hot pan and cook for 2-3 minutes or until they turn pink.

Add the coconut milk to the shrimp and simmer for 3-5 minutes.

Taste the sauce and add seasoning as desired.

Serve over the rice.

1 cup basmati rice

2 Roma tomatoes, diced

1 tablespoon cilantro, chopped

1 pound raw shelled shrimp

1 tablespoon curry powder

Sea salt and black pepper to taste

1 teaspoon cayenne pepper (optional)

2 tablespoons extra virgin olive oil

1 cup condensed coconut milk

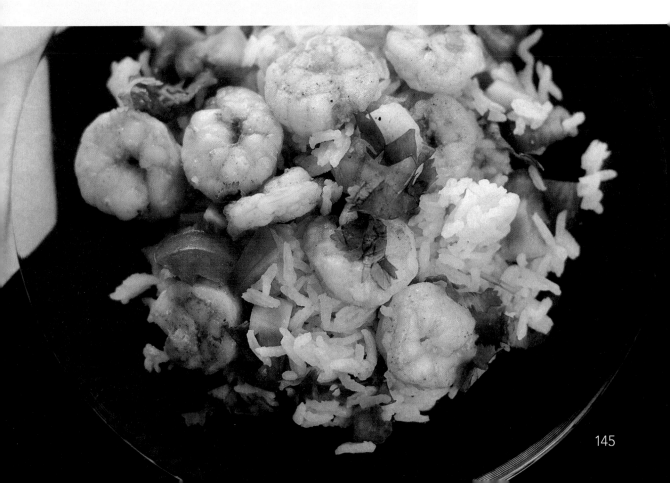

turkey burgers
with fig jam

Serves 4

1 pound organic ground turkey

¼ cup green onions

¼ cup organic Italian seasoned breadcrumbs

1 tablespoon garlic powder

1 teaspoon sea salt

¼ teaspoon black pepper

Fig & Onion Marmalade:

1 large sweet Vidalia onion, thinly sliced

4 dried figs, cut into quarters

2 tablespoons balsamic vinegar

Honey-Goat Cheese Spread:

1 small log organic goat cheese

1 tablespoon raw or local honey

Pretzel or sprouted grain buns for serving

Heat grill to medium high heat. Meanwhile, combine turkey burger ingredients and form into four patties. Once grill is hot, add turkey burgers and cook 5-7 minutes per side.

Heat a large skillet over medium heat and cook onions until caramelized, about 10 minutes.

Add figs and balsamic vinegar to onions and turn heat to low. Cook for an additional 10 minutes.

In a small bowl, mix together goat cheese and honey.

 Warm buns in oven or on grill before serving.

Remove turkey burgers from grill and let cool for 5 minutes.

To assemble burgers, spread honey goat cheese on bottom of the bun, top with fig and onion marmalade. Place turkey burger on top.

Serve with veggie ribbon salad if desired.

tip▶ Try swapping out pretzel bun for a portobello bun. Simply, drizzle both sides of portabella mushrooms with olive oil and salt and pepper and grill for 5 minutes each side.

veggie burgers

Makes 8-10 burgers

Preheat oven to 375°F.

Add Brussels sprouts, mushrooms and broccoli or cauliflower to a food processor and pulse to chop.

Add all ingredients, except eggs to a large bowl and mix well with your hands.

Add eggs and mix to combine.

Form mixture into burger patties and set aside on a plate. Cover and put in the refrigerator for 30 minutes to set.

Preheat grill pan or skillet to medium high heat and drizzle pan with extra virgin olive oil. When pan is hot, add burgers and cook on each side for 3-4 minutes or until nicely browned. Burgers may fall apart a bit when you flip—simply re-mold by pressing down on burgers to flatten.

Place grill pan or skillet in the oven and cook for 10-15 minutes. Let cool before serving. Add to your favorite burger bun or place on a bed of mixed greens and enjoy.

Top with sliced avocado if desired.

1 cup organic long grain rice, cooked in chicken broth

1 cup Brussels sprouts, stems removed and sliced

1 cup mushrooms

1 cup broccoli or cauliflower florets

½ cup green onion, finely chopped

¼ cup fresh basil, finely chopped

1 cup organic tomato sauce

1 tablespoon garlic powder

Sea Salt & Black Pepper to taste

2 eggs, beaten

pesto crusted salmon

Serves 4

4 6-ounce salmon fillets

2 garlic cloves

1 cup broccoli florets

¼ cup extra virgin olive oil plus 2 tablespoons, separated

¼ cup parmesan cheese, grated

¼ cup unsalted shelled pistachios

tip▶ May use this broccoli pesto recipe as a stuffing for chicken or steak pinwheels. Simply pound out individual pieces of chicken or steak using a meat mallet, add a spoonful of pesto to the center of each and roll into a pinwheel and secure with a toothpick. Sprinkle with salt and pepper and pan fry pinwheels until browned. Finish in the oven until fully cooked.

Preheat the oven to 375°F.

Rub both sides of salmon fillets with 1 tablespoon olive oil.

Combine the rest of the ingredients and pulse in a food processor until mixture turns to a chunky purée. Season to taste with sea salt and black pepper. Coat the top of the salmon with the mixture.

Add 1 tablespoon extra virgin olive oil to a cast-iron skillet or non-stick pan over medium heat on the stove top. Place salmon skin side down for 2-3 minutes until skin is sizzling.

Place the pan on the middle oven rack and bake for 8-10 minutes or until the salmon looks flaky and the pesto turns golden brown.

> The base of your typical pesto is basil. Swap the basil broccoli to bump up the nutrition.

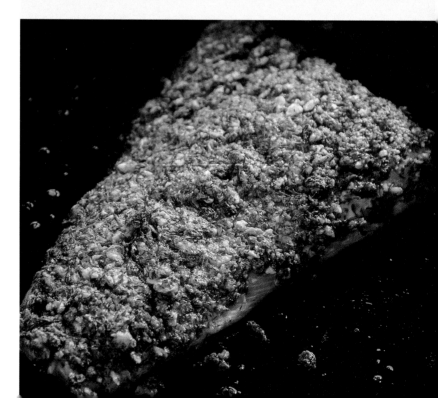

chilean sea bass
with miso broth

Serves 4

Add rice, water, celery and onions to a large pot and cook according to package directions, about 15-20 minutes.

Meanwhile, add miso broth*, celery leaves and ginger to a large pot and bring to a medium, low boil. Pat sea bass dry with paper towel. Season both sides of sea bass with salt and pepper.

Add 1 tablespoon extra virgin olive oil to a large skillet and heat over medium high heat. Place sea bass, skin side up in pan and cook for 4-5 minutes until nicely browned. Flip and cook 4 minutes or more. Fish should flake with a fork. Remove miso broth from heat. Season with sea salt if needed.

To serve, add one cup of spinach to a wide, deep bowl. Add a heaping spoonful of warm rice over spinach and top with sea bass fillet. Spoon miso broth over spinach, rice and fillet. Add a few drops of toasted sesame oil over dish and garnish with green onions and sesame seeds.

1 cup of white jasmine rice

2 cups of water

½ cup of celery, chopped

½ cup of onions, chopped

4 cups of miso broth

1 tablespoon Bragg's Liquid Aminos

2 large bunches of celery leaves

1 tablespoon fresh ginger, grated

4 (4 ounce) Chilean sea bass fillets

4 cups of baby spinach

Toasted sesame oil for topping

4 green onions, chopped

Sesame seeds for garnish

tip▶ Miso broth can be found in the soup aisle near the other broth/stocks. If miso broth is not available, make your own by using organic miso paste and water.

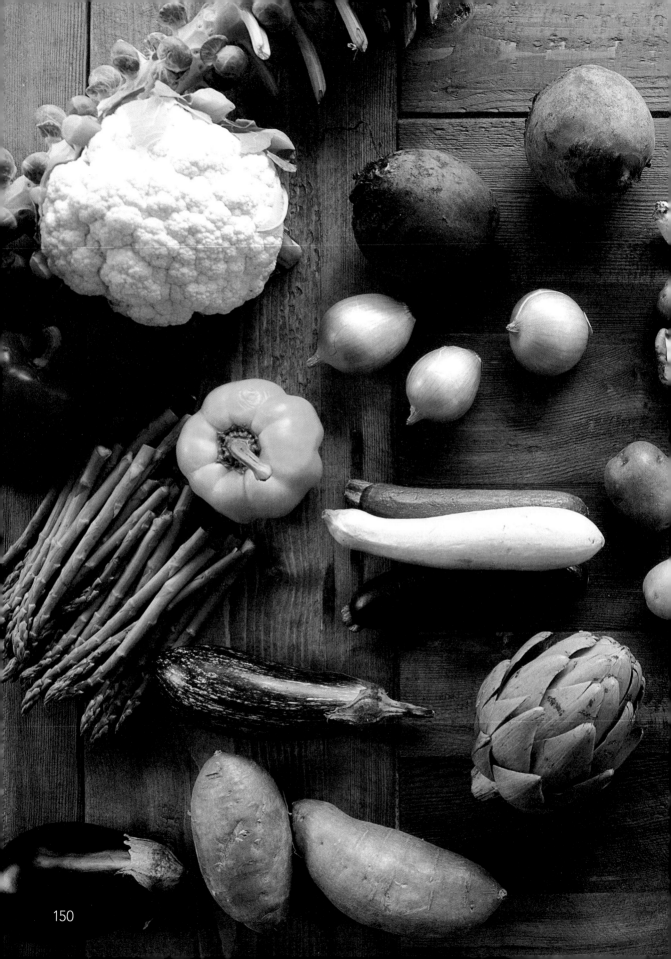

sides

not so candied pecans

2 cups raw pecans

2 tablespoon honey

1 tablespoon agave nectar

Pinch sea salt

Preheat oven to 350 degrees F.

Lay pecans evenly on a parchment lined baking sheet.

Bake for 10 minutes until pecans are lightly toasted.

Combine with honey, agave nectar and a pinch of sea salt, then drizzle on the hot pecans. Toss lightly and spread evenly on pan.

Bake for an additional 5 minutes.

Let cool for 20-30 minutes then break pecans apart to serve. Can be stored at room temperature for up to a week.

maple glazed carrots & leeks

¼ cup virgin coconut oil, melted

1 tablespoon maple syrup

¼ teaspoon sea salt

¼ teaspoon cayenne pepper

6 medium carrots, peeled

3 large stalks of leeks, sliced

¼ cup parsley, chopped

Serves 4

Preheat oven to 375°F.

Combine virgin coconut oil, maple syrup, salt, and cayenne in a small bowl and whisk to mix.

Cut the carrots in half and slice lengthwise. Slice and clean leeks. Combine carrots and leeks on a baking sheet. Cover with virgin coconut oil mixture and toss to coat.

Place baking sheet in oven and cook for 20-25 minutes or until tender. Remove from oven and top with parsley before serving.

tip▶ To clean leeks, cut off and discard the dark green leaves an inch or so above the white part. Slice white part; rinse in a colander under cold water.

roasted brussels sprouts

Serves 4

Preheat the oven to 375°F.

Cut off the stem end of the Brussels sprouts and cut in half. Place the halved sprouts in a bowl and combine all the ingredients.

Place the sprouts on a cooking sheet and bake for 40-50 minutes. They should be golden brown and slightly crispy.

1½ pounds Brussels sprouts

2 tablespoons extra virgin olive oil

½ teaspoon sea salt

¼ teaspoon black pepper

2 garlic cloves, diced

Drizzle balsamic vinegar (optional)

tip ▶ Any vegetable can be roasted in the oven. Try broccoli, cauliflower, or asparagus. Easy and delicious!

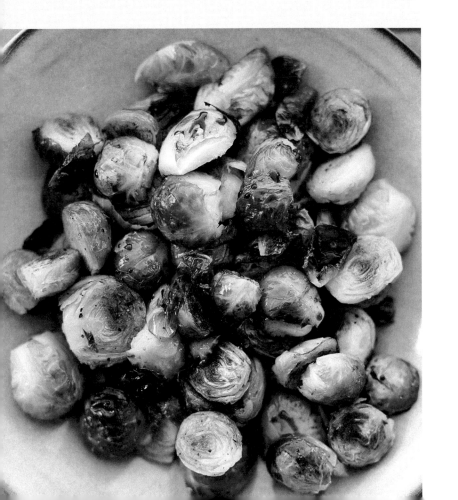

roasted root vegetables

2 parsnips, cut into 1-inch pieces

2 large carrots, sliced

1 large sweet potato, cut into 1-inch pieces

2 purple potatoes, cut into 1-inch pieces

2 large yellow potatoes, cut into 1-inch pieces

2 tablespoons extra virgin olive oil

Sea salt & black pepper

1 tablespoon dried thyme

Preheat oven to 375°F.

Place all of the chopped vegetables on a large baking sheet.

Toss vegetables with olive oil, salt, and black pepper, and thyme.

Bake in oven for 30-45 minutes.

oven roasted beets

Serves 4

4 large or 8 small beets, peeled and sliced into circles

2 tablespoons extra virgin olive oil

Sea salt & black pepper

Preheat oven to 375°F.

Spread 1 tablespoon of olive oil on a large baking sheet.

Arrange beet slices on oiled baking sheet in a single layer.

Drizzle remaining 1 tablespoon olive oil on beet slices.

Season with sea salt and black pepper.

Bake in oven for 30 minutes until slightly crispy around the edges.

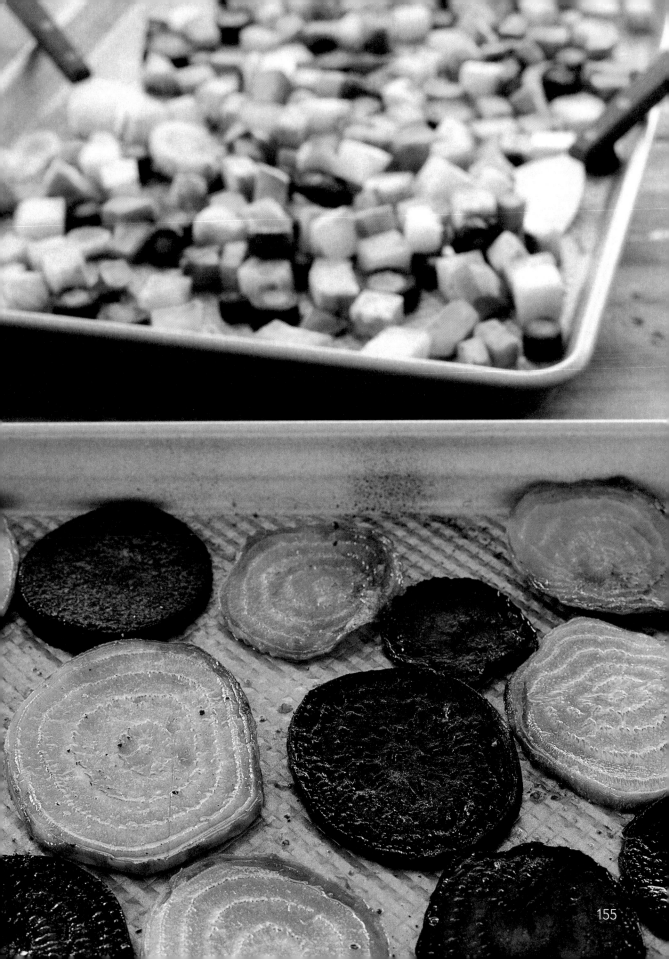

For the crust:

¾ cup walnuts

1¼ cups whole wheat pastry flour, plus more for dusting

1¼ cups quinoa or almond flour

2 tablespoons fresh thyme or rosemary, chopped

¾ teaspoon sea salt

¾ teaspoon black pepper

¼ cup extra virgin olive oil

¼ cup virgin coconut oil

7 tablespoons ice cold water

For the filling:

1½ pounds sweet potato, peeled and sliced

2 tablespoons extra virgin olive oil

½ teaspoon sea salt

¼ cup red or sweet onions, sliced and separated into rings

1 cup shredded cheddar cheese

1 large egg white mixed with 1 teaspoon water

1 teaspoon chopped fresh thyme or rosemary depending on what you chose for the crust

tip ▶ To resemble the Food Target and cover photo, use broccoli, yellow peppers, sweet potatoes, and red peppers to resemble the Food Target colors. Vegetables can be lightly cooked before assembling on the tart. Follow recipe instructions.

sweet potato tart

Serves 4-6

Preheat oven to 425°F.

To make the crust:

Prepare crust by placing walnuts in a food processor and pulse until finely ground. Add flours, thyme, sea salt, and black pepper, and pulse to combine. Add the solid virgin coconut oil and pulse until crumbly. Drizzle olive oil and ice water until mixture is combined. The dough will seem wetter than usual. Wrap the dough in plastic wrap and store in refrigerator for 15 minutes or up to 2 days.

To make the filling:

Toss the sweet potatoes with 1 tablespoon of olive oil, and season with sea salt and black pepper. Spread on two-thirds of a large cookie sheet. Toss the onions with 1 teaspoon of olive oil and season with sea salt and black pepper. Spread on remaining one-third of the cookie sheet. Roast in the oven for 10 minutes. Remove from the oven to cool slightly. Reduce oven temperature to 375°F.

Place dough on a floured nonstick baking mat or parchment paper. Dust the top of the dough with flour and roll into a 15-inch circle. Place the dough on the baking mat or parchment on a cookie sheet.

Sprinkle cheese on the crust, leaving a 2-inch border. Place the sweet potatoes in two overlapping rings over the outside edge of the cheese.

Place the onions in a ring just inside those two sweet potatoes rows. Use remaining sweet potatoes to fill in an overlapping ring in the center.

Pick up the edges of the crust to form small pleats. Brush with the egg whites. Drizzle olive oil over the top of the tart and sprinkle with remaining thyme or rosemary.

Bake the tart for 40-45 minutes or until lightly browned and cooked through. Cool for 10 minutes before slicing.

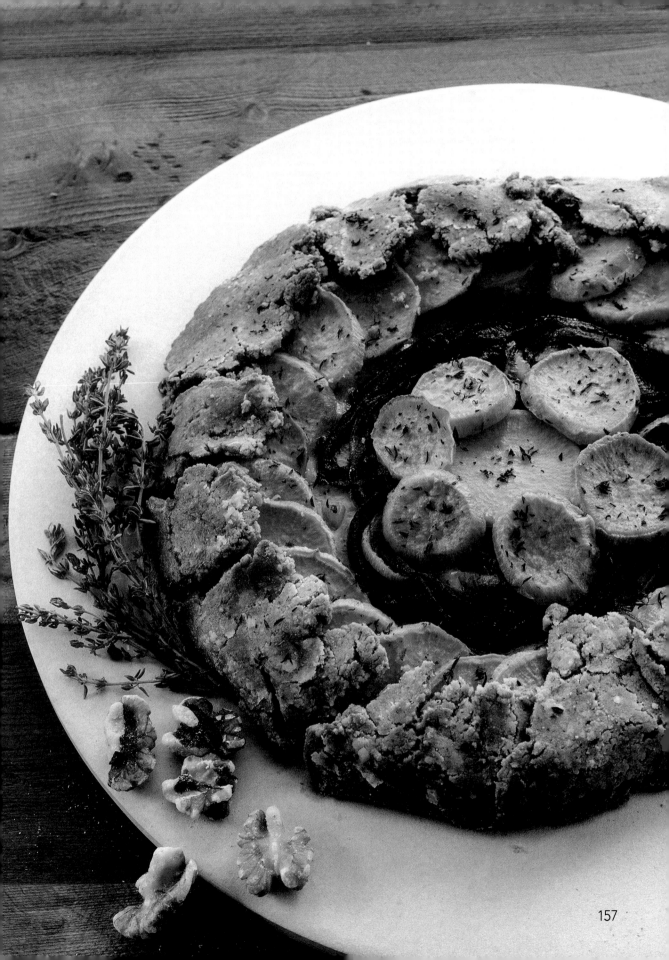

sweet potato fries

Serves 4

1 pound potatoes of choice, scrubbed clean, dried and cut into fries

1½ tablespoons extra virgin olive oil

Sea salt & black pepper to taste

Adjust oven rack to middle position and heat oven to 425°F.

Toss potatoes and olive oil on cookie sheet. Season with sea salt and black pepper and toss again to blend.

Spread potatoes out into a single layer.

Cook for 15 minutes; turn using metal spatula.

Return pan to oven and cook 10-15 minutes more until the potatoes begin to brown and get crunchy.

tip ▶ These fries can be made with red skin potatoes, sweet potatoes, or even root vegetables.

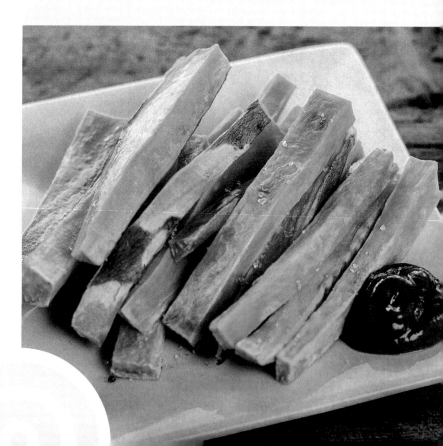

baked red skin potato chips

Serves 4

Heat oven to 425°F.

Line a baking sheet with parchment paper.

Cut red skin potatoes into thin slices using a mandolin or sharp knife. Spread on baking sheet and toss well with extra virgin olive oil. Arrange potato slices evenly on the baking sheet. Sprinkle with salt, pepper or your favorite seasoning. Bake for 40-45 minutes or until crispy.

*No need to flip—potatoes will get crispy on both sides. To speed up the process, heat oven to 450°F and bake for 30-35 minutes.

Serve with dill pickle dip if desired - Combine all ingredients in a small food processor and mix well. Season to taste with salt and pepper.

1 pound red skin potatoes

2 tablespoons extra virgin olive oil

Dill Pickle Dip:

8-ounce container organic cream cheese

5.3-ounce container organic grass-fed plain yogurt

2 tablespoons green onions, chopped

2 tablespoons dill pickles, chopped

½ teaspoon garlic powder

½ teaspoon onion powder

½ teaspoon dried dill

Salt and pepper to taste

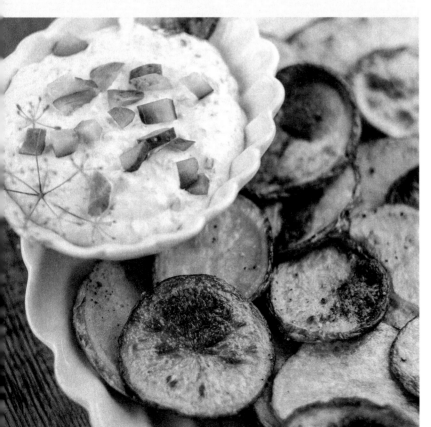

kristen:
During my pregnancy I was obsessed with pickles and decided to come up with a dip that could curb my cravings.

asian broccoli salad

Serves 4

3 cups broccoli florets

¼ cup shredded carrots

2 green onions, chopped

¼ cup roasted and salted sunflower seeds

1 tablespoon sesame seeds

Combine broccoli, green onions, sunflower seeds and sesame seeds in a large bowl.

In a small food processor, mix all dressing ingredients until combined. Add more water to thin if needed.

Add dressing to broccoli mixture and toss to mix.

tip▶ Extra dressing can be used as salad dressing, a dip for chicken or beef, or drizzled on vegetables or potatoes.

Dressing:

¼ cup natural peanut butter

1 tablespoon freshly grated ginger

1 tablespoons Bragg's Liquid Aminos (low sodium non-GMO soy sauce)

1 tablespoon brown rice wine vinegar

1 teaspoon raw honey

1 teaspoon sesame oil

¼ cup warm water

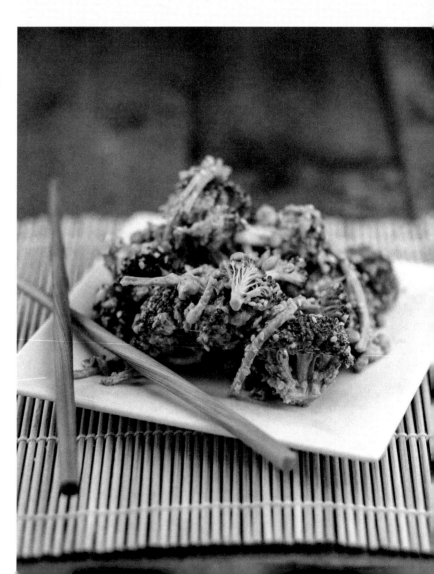

mashed cauliflower

Serves 4 (pictured on page 111)

Place cauliflower and broth in a large pot. Cover partially with lid, allowing steam to escape.

Cook on medium heat until cauliflower is soft.

Mash with a potato masher, then mix in parmesan cheese and season with sea salt and black pepper.

1 large head cauliflower, chopped into florets

1 cup chicken or vegetable broth

Sea salt & black pepper to taste

Freshly grated parmesan cheese

 Mashed cauliflower has the same creamy texture as mashed potatoes but is much lower in calories which means you can go for seconds and not feel guilty! This cruciferous vegetable also contains fiber, vitamins, and minerals.

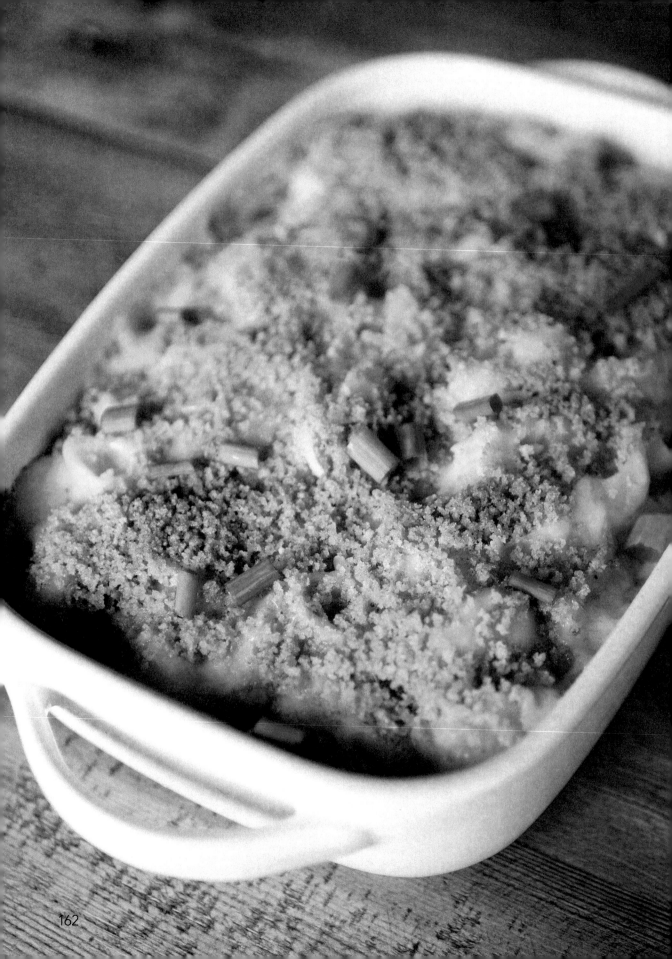

butternut squash mac & cheese

Serves 6

Preheat oven to 350°F.

Spread squash on parchment lined baking sheet and drizzle with extra virgin olive oil. Sprinkle with sea salt and black pepper. Bake for 20 minutes until tender.

Meanwhile, create a roux with ½ cup of butter, flour and milk by melting the butter over medium low heat. Add flour and mix with a whisk. Turn heat to medium and slowly add in milk using whisk to incorporate all ingredients. Sauce should thicken after 2-3 minutes. Remove from heat.

Once squash is cooked, add to a food processor with 1 teaspoon sea salt and puree. Add squash puree and cheese to roux. Season to taste with salt and pepper.

Bring a large pot of salted water to boil. Add pasta to boiling water and cook according to package instructions. Drain pasta, return to pot and add in squash roux and green onions. Mix well.

For topping, heat reserved 2 tablespoons butter in a skillet over medium heat and add breadcrumbs and ½ teaspoon of salt. Cook for 2-3 minutes. Set aside.

Grease a large casserole dish with cooking spray and add in pasta mixture. Top with reserved ½ cup of topping.

Cover with foil and bake for 20 minutes. Uncover and cook for an additional 10 minutes. Turn oven to medium broil and cook for 2-3 minutes or until breadcrumbs are lightly browned. Remove from oven and let sit for 5 minutes before serving.

4 cups butternut squash (fresh, pre-cut works best)

1 pound pasta shells (large pasta shells work best)

¼ organic grass-fed salted butter + 2 tablespoons reserved

½ cup organic all-purpose flour

2 cups organic whole milk or unsweetened coconut milk

8-ounce block organic cheddar cheese, shredded (reserve ½ cup for topping)

Organic panko breadcrumbs

½ cup green onions, chopped

tip ▶ Adding butternut squash puree provides a creamy consistency and delicious flavor with a punch of nutrition. Plus, this recipe is kid-approved!

zucchini & squash casserole

Serves 6

2 medium zucchini or summer squash, sliced (can use a combination)

1 large onion, sliced and pulled into individual rings

2 large tomatoes, peeled and sliced

½ cup parmesan cheese, grated

Sea salt & black pepper to taste

Preheat oven to 400°F.

Grease a large, deep casserole dish with extra virgin olive oil.

In order, evenly layer half of the zucchini, onion, tomato, and cheese into casserole dish.

Drizzle with olive oil and sprinkle with sea salt and black pepper.

Repeat order a second time with remaining half of the ingredients.

Bake covered for 45 minutes. Remove cover and cook an additional 15 minutes until cheese is slightly golden brown.

Let sit for 10-15 minutes before serving.

kristen: *We became masters at making this recipe after watching our Grammy make this with love and perfection many times on our summer vacations Up North.*

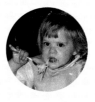

veggie pesto wraps

Makes 4 Wraps

Slice summer squash, zucchini and portabellas into slices lengthwise. Toss with extra virgin olive oil and salt and pepper.

Preheat grill pan or grill to medium heat and cook vegetables for 2-3 minutes per side or until tender and grill marks form.

Meanwhile, combine all broccoli pesto ingredients in a food processor and blend to mix. Season to taste with sea salt.

To assemble wraps, start by spreading an even layer of broccoli pesto over the wraps and top with cooked vegetables, sun dried tomatoes, and fresh mozzarella.

Roll up tightly and serve.

1 large summer squash

1 large zucchini

4 large portabella mushroom caps

1 jar sun dried tomatoes

4 slices fresh mozzarella

1 package spinach or sprouted grain wraps

Broccoli Pesto

1 cup broccoli florets

2 garlic cloves, chopped

¼ cup parmesan cheese, grated

¼ cup salted, shelled pistachios

¼ cup extra virgin olive oil

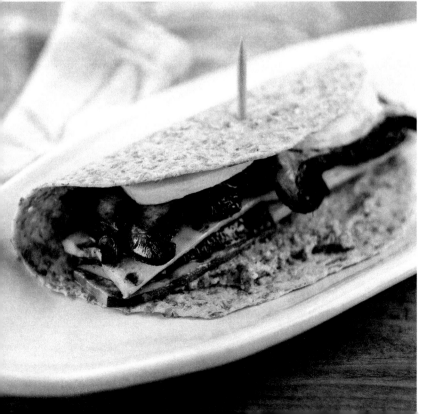

tip▶ May also use your favorite bread or ciabatta loaf to make veggie pesto sandwiches.

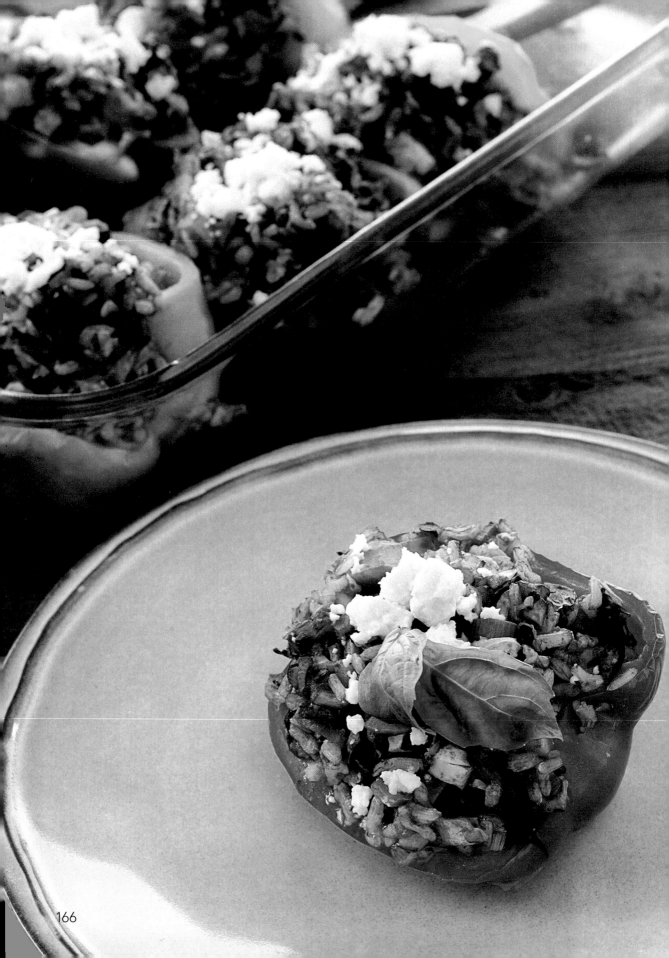

veggie stuffed peppers

Serves 6

Preheat oven to 375°F.

In a small pot, bring broth to a boil and add in rice. Once rice mixture begins to boil, cover and cook on a low simmer for 40-45 minutes.

Remove from heat and set aside to cool slightly.

Slice peppers in half and remove seeds and stems.

Place peppers cut side up on a lightly greased 9x13 inch baking dish.

In a large bowl combine rice and the remaining ingredients except cheese, and spoon mixture into peppers.

Cover baking dish with foil and cook for 30 minutes. Remove foil and top stuffed peppers with cheese.

Bake uncovered for an additional 15 minutes. Let cool for 5 minutes and serve.

1 cup organic brown rice

2 cups organic chicken broth

3 bell peppers

½ cup asparagus, chopped

½ cup Brussels sprouts, stems removed and sliced

½ cup mushrooms, chopped

½ cup broccoli florets

½ cup cauliflower florets

½ cup green onion, finely chopped

¼ cup basil, finely chopped

2 cloves garlic, minced

1 cup organic marinara sauce

½ cup feta or goat cheese, crumbled

fried rice

Serves 4

1½ cups organic brown basmati rice

2-3 eggs

½ cup diced carrots

½ cup diced onion

½ cup frozen peas

1 tablespoon extra virgin olive oil

1 tablespoon roasted sesame seeds

½ teaspoon black pepper

½ teaspoon sea salt

1 tablespoons Bragg's Liquid Aminos or low sodium soy sauce

1 teaspoon toasted sesame oil

Garnish with chopped green onions

Cook rice according to package directions. Rinse cooked rice in a strainer, and set aside to cool and dry slightly.

Scramble the eggs lightly in a small frying pan. They will continue to cook slightly when added into the rice. Set aside.

Heat the olive oil in a large frying pan over medium high heat. When the oil is very hot, add the onions and carrots. Stir constantly so that the vegetables don't burn.

When the onions and carrots are soft, add the peas and rice, and mix together. Cook for 5 minutes.

Chop the scrambled eggs and add them to the rice. Stir to combine.

Season with salt and black pepper. Sprinkle in the sesame seeds.

Add the sesame oil and Bragg's and cook for 3 more minutes.

tip▶ Serve this dish hot with any Asian inspired entrée. To make a one-dish entrée, add diced, cooked chicken, beef, or shrimp.

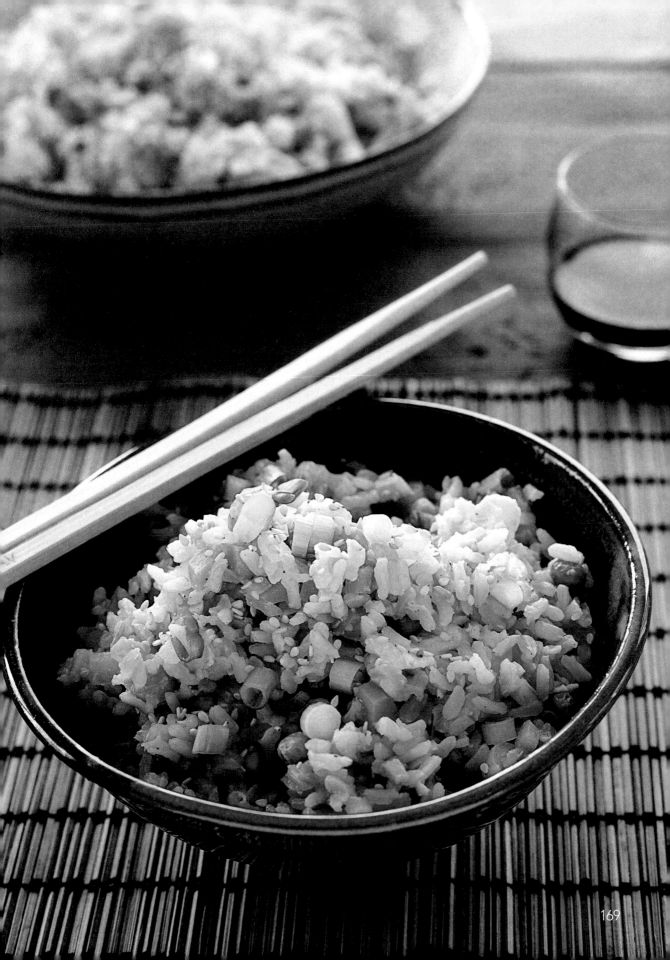

greek farro

Serves 6

2 cups farro

4 cups water chicken broth

2 large tomatoes, chopped

½ cup cucumbers, chopped

¼ cup red onion, diced

¼ cup Greek olives, sliced

½ cup fresh basil, chopped

½ cup fresh parsley, chopped

¼ cup balsamic vinegar

¼ cup extra virgin olive oil

Salt & pepper to taste

Feta cheese, crumbled for topper

Add farro and water or broth to a large sauce pot. Bring to a boil, cover, and reduce heat to simmer.

Cook for 15 minutes or until farro is cooked and most of the liquid is absorbed. Drain if necessary.

Add cooked farro to a large mixing bowl and add remaining ingredients.

Toss to mix .

Top with crumbled feta cheese.

tip▶ Serve this salad warm or chilled. It's especially great leftover with a fried egg on top.

 Farro is one of the oldest grains cultivated by humans and is a great source of both protein and fiber.

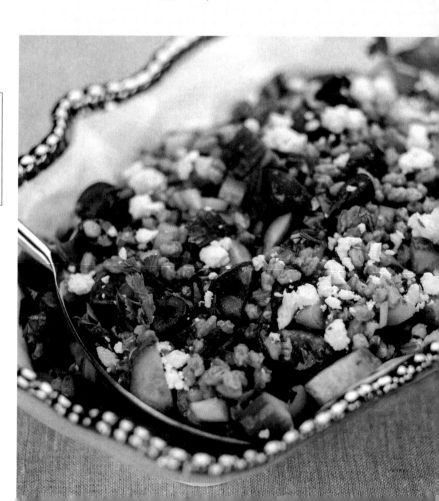

dad's favorite potato salad

Serves 6

Preheat over to 425°F.

Line a baking sheet with parchment paper and spread potatoes evenly over sheet. Drizzle with extra virgin olive oil and salt and pepper.

Bake for 20-25 minutes or until brown and crispy. Remove from oven and let cool.

Combine potatoes and remaining ingredients in a large bowl. Mix well and store in the refrigerator 1 hour or overnight before serving.

3 pounds red skin potatoes, chopped

4 stalks celery, chopped

4 organic dill pickles, chopped

4 green onions, chopped

6 hard boiled eggs, chopped

½ cup avocado oil mayonnaise

2 tablespoons Dijon mustard

2 tablespoons dried or fresh dill

Salt and pepper to taste

pearl couscous
& figs

Serves 4

1 cups black mission figs, diced

1 cup tricolor pearled couscous

3 green onions, white and green parts, sliced thin

½ cup pistachios, chopped

¼ cup parsley, chopped

2 tablespoons extra virgin olive oil

2 tablespoons lemon juice

Sea salt & black pepper

Place diced figs in a bowl and add ¼ cup boiling water. Cover with plastic wrap and set aside to soften.

Cook couscous according to package directions. Put cooked couscous in a serving bowl.

Drain the water from the figs and add them to the couscous.

Add the green onions, pistachios, and parsley.

Add olive oil and lemon juice, and season with salt and black pepper to taste.

tip ▶ Can be served chilled.

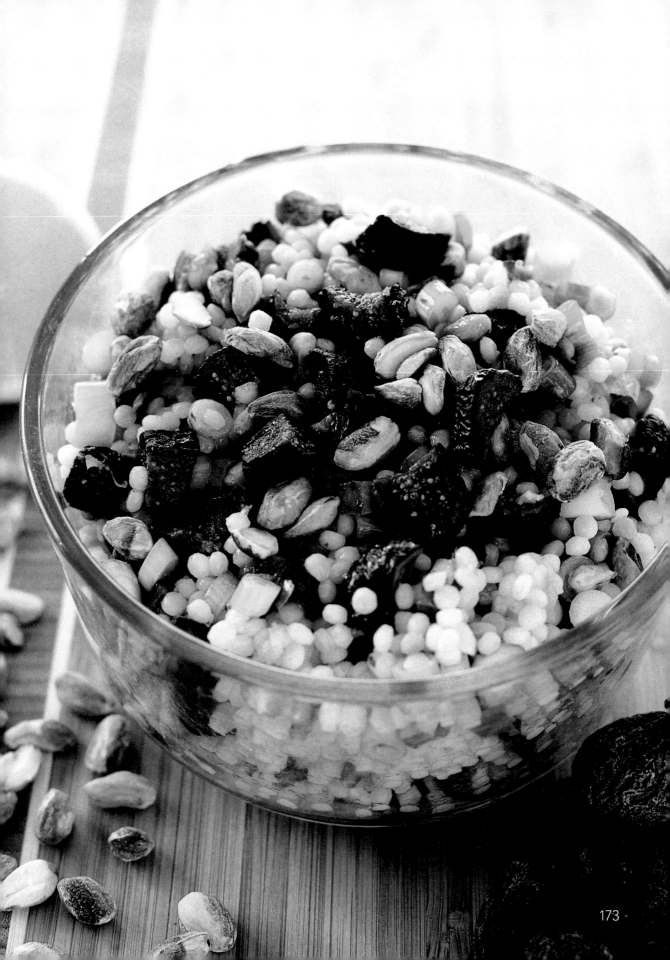

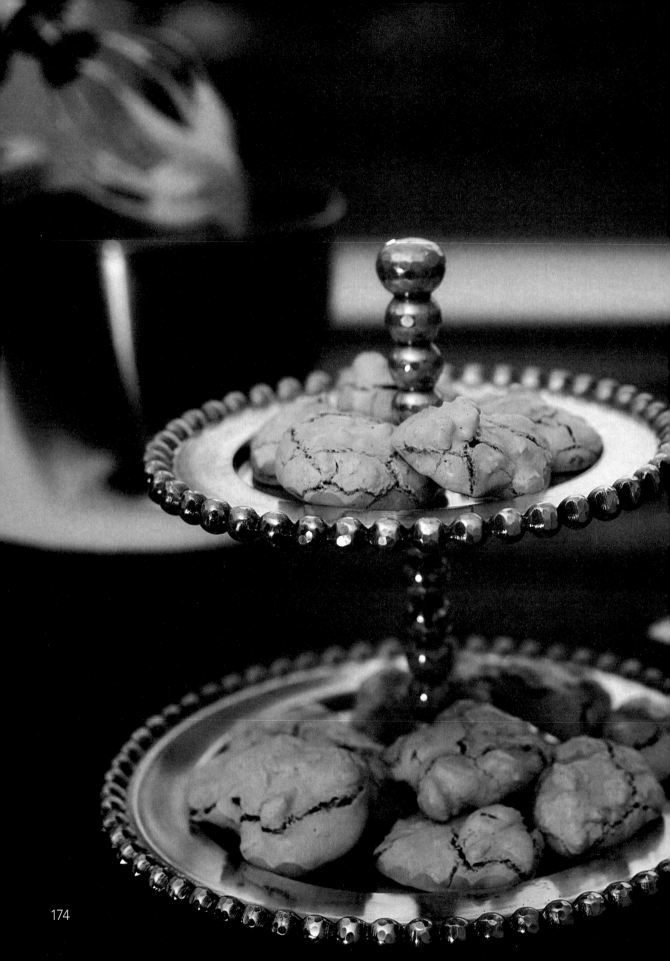

desserts

meringue date cookies

Makes 24 cookies

3 egg whites, room temperature

¼ teaspoon sea salt

1¾ cups powdered sugar

1 teaspoon flour

1 cup pecans, broken

1 cup pitted dates, chopped

1 teaspoon vanilla extract

Preheat oven to 300°F.

Add salt to egg whites and beat to a stiff foam.

Sift together powdered sugar and flour. Add one tablespoon at a time to the egg whites, mixing thoroughly between each addition. Continue beating until very stiff. Fold in nuts, dates, and vanilla.

Drop from teaspoon onto cookie sheet lined with parchment paper.

Bake for 30 minutes.

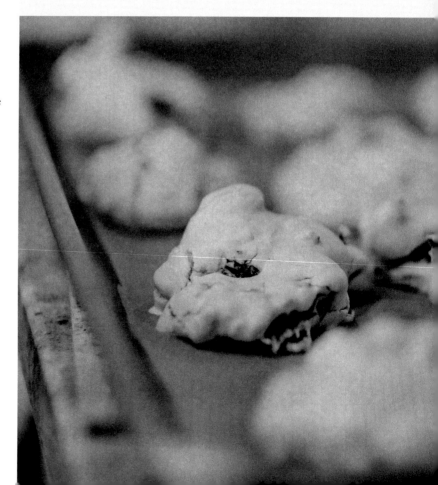

kristen: *These cookies are a Holiday favorite passed down from our Great Grandma Kramer. Grandpa "Gido" is the official taste tester with the same response every year. "Mmmmm... these are better than last year." We share this family recipe with you because we would hate for anyone to miss out on this delicious experience.*

176

hot cacao

Serves 1

Combine all ingredients in a blender and mix until frothy and delicious.

8 ounces warmed water, coconut or almond milk

1 tablespoon cacao powder

2 teaspoons raw or local honey

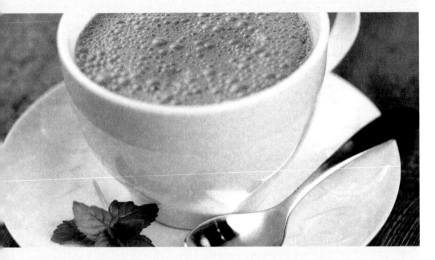

buckeye bark

Makes 15-20 pieces

Line a cookie sheet with waxed paper.

Melt 1 bag of chocolate chips in a double boiler. Spread the melted chocolate in a thin layer over waxed paper lined cookie sheet. Place in freezer for 10 minutes to harden.

Mix crunchy almond or peanut butter with agave nectar and vanilla extract.

Remove melted chocolate from freezer and spread nut butter mixture evenly over the top. Place in freezer for another 5 minutes to harden.

Melt the 2nd bag of chocolate chips and spread on top of frozen nut butter mixture. Return to freezer for 1 hour.

Once chocolate peanut butter mixture is hardened, break into medium-sized pieces and serve.

2 bags dark chocolate chips

1 jar crunchy almond or peanut butter

1 tablespoon agave nectar

1 tablespoon vanilla extract

tip ▶ Choose nut butters that have one ingredient. Example: peanuts.

177

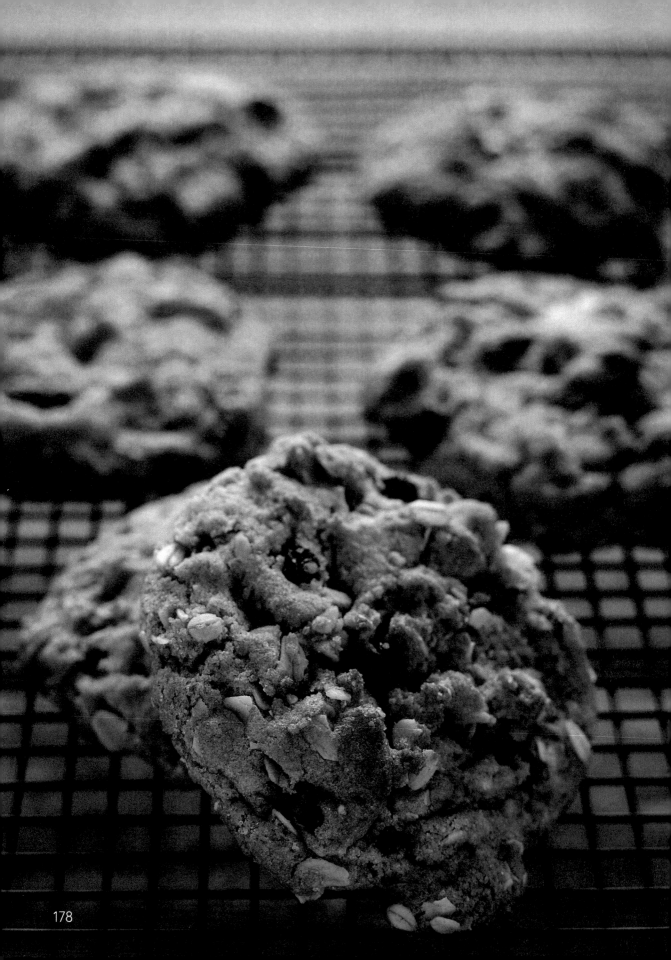

holly's oatmeal raisin cookies

Makes 12 Cookies

Preheat oven to 350°F.

Whisk together the eggs and vanilla. Add the raisins and cover for 1 hour, allowing raisins to become soft.

In medium bowl, sift together the flour, cinnamon, and baking soda.

Cream together the butter, virgin coconut oil, and sugars. Add flour mixture and combine (mix will seem dry). Mix in the egg and raisin mixture. Finally, add in oatmeal and combine.

Grease a cookie sheet with virgin coconut oil and drop the dough in ¼ cup balls 2 inches apart. Flatten each ball slightly using your palm.

Bake 10-12 minutes in the preheated oven, or until golden brown. Cool slightly, remove from sheet to wire rack. Cool completely.

2 eggs

1 teaspoon vanilla extract

1 cup raisins

1⅔ cup all-purpose flour

1 teaspoon cinnamon

2 teaspoons baking soda

⅓ cup unsalted butter (room temperature)

⅓ cup virgin coconut oil at room temperature (should not be liquid)

⅔ cup brown sugar

⅔ cup white sugar

1⅓ cup rolled oats

holly: *Matt is a fabulous cook and loves to create new recipes, but he doesn't like to bake because he'd rather experiment than follow precise directions. Luckily, baking is my passion, so we make a great team!*

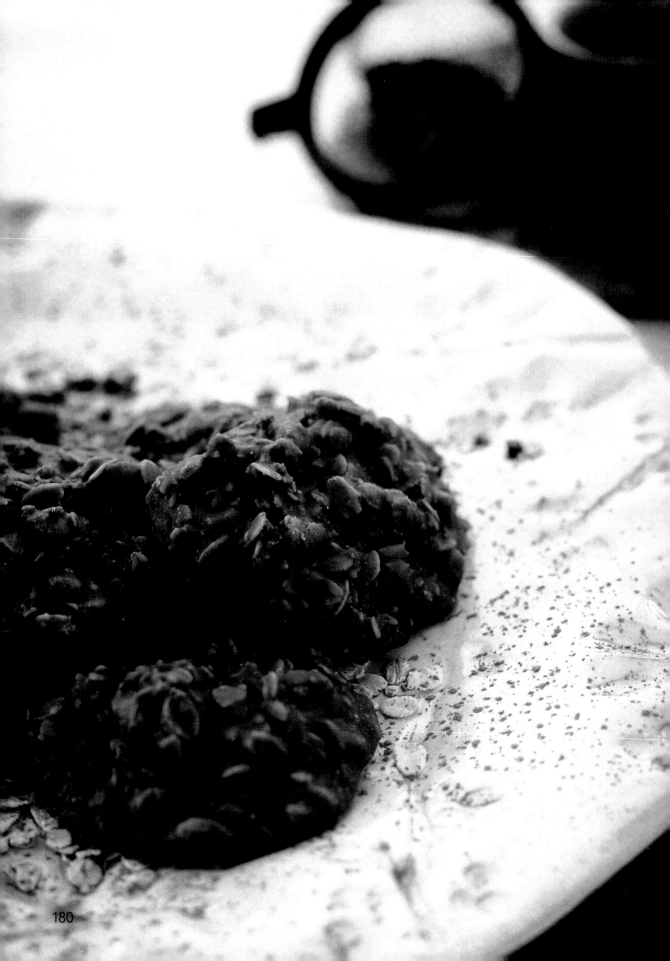

no-bake cookies

Makes 12 cookies

Heat cocoa, sugar, milk, butter, and virgin coconut oil over medium heat. Heat these very, very slowly to a boil. Boil them for no longer than 90-120 seconds and remove from heat.

Mix together oats, peanut butter, and vanilla with a big wooden spoon or mixer.

Pour the hot mix over the oatmeal mix. Stir together for 4 minutes to allow oats to absorb liquid.

Using a large mixing spoon, drop spoonfuls on wax paper and let cool.

3 tablespoons unsweetened cocoa powder

2 cups cane sugar

½ cup skim milk

¼ cup butter

¼ cup virgin coconut oil

3 cups rolled oats

½ cup natural peanut butter

1 tablespoon vanilla extract

trail mix treats

Combine nuts, seeds, and dried fruit and set aside.

Melt 1 bag of dark chocolate chips over a double boiler.

Line a baking tray with waxed paper. Using a ladle, drop small dollops of melted chocolate on the waxed paper.

Sprinkle chocolate with trail mixture and let cool.

¼ cup pumpkin seeds

¼ cup whole almonds

¼ cup dried cranberries or cherries

¼ cup raisins

1 bag dark chocolate chips

tip ▶ For convenience, choose store-bought trail mix combinations that include raw nuts, and dried fruits without added oil or sugar.

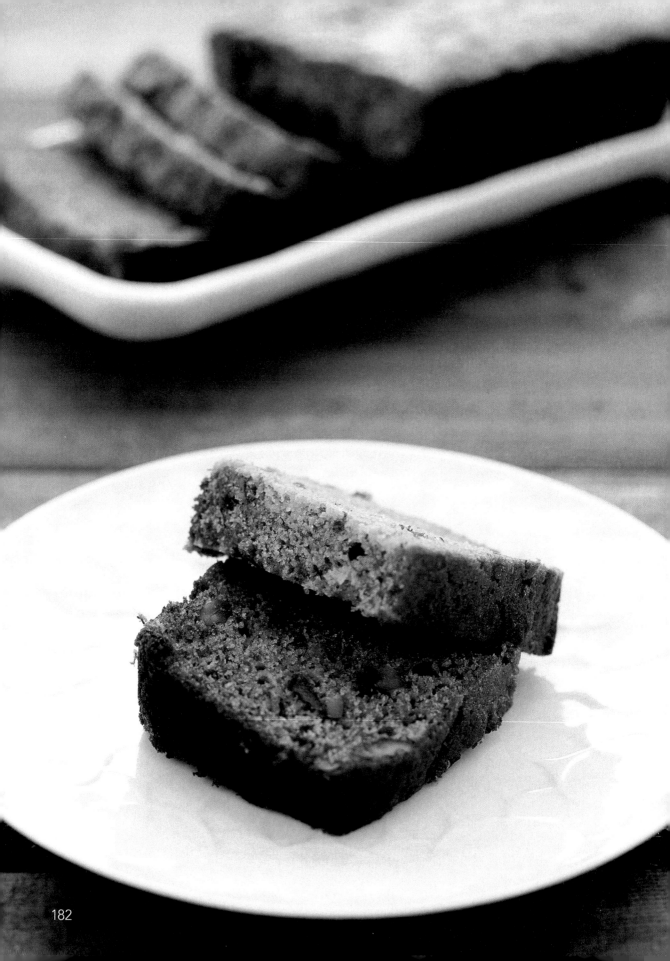

banana bread

Serves 10-12

Preheat oven to 325°F.

Beat together the sugar and eggs on medium until light and fluffy, roughly 5 minutes.

Very slowly, drizzle in the oil, still beating the mixture on medium. Then add the applesauce and continue mixing.

Add the banana, Greek Yogurt, honey, and vanilla. Mix together on low speed until combined.

Combine the flour, baking soda, cinnamon, and sea salt, and fold into the banana mixture until thoroughly combined. Stir in the toasted walnuts.

Pour the batter into a greased 9x5 inch loaf pan.

Bake for 50-55 minutes, until toothpick comes out clean.

½ cup white sugar

2 eggs

¼ cup and 1 tablespoon virgin coconut oil (melted)

¼ cup applesauce

3½ ripe bananas, mashed with a fork to remove all lumps

2 tablespoons plain Greek yogurt

½ cup plus 2 teaspoons honey

1 teaspoon vanilla extract

1½ cups whole wheat flour

1 teaspoon baking soda

¼ teaspoon cinnamon

½ teaspoon sea salt

¾ cup walnuts, toasted

This is a healthy spin on your traditional banana bread. It makes for a great gift from the kitchen.

chocolate chip peanut butter banana bread

Serves 10-12

1 cup white whole wheat flour

⅓ cup pure cane sugar

⅓ cup brown sugar, packed

1 teaspoon baking powder

½ teaspoon baking soda

¼ teaspoon sea salt

3 very ripe bananas, mashed

⅓ cup natural crunchy peanut butter

2 tablespoons plain nonfat Greek yogurt

1 large egg

1 teaspoon vanilla extract

2 tablespoons virgin coconut oil

¾ cup dark chocolate chips

Preheat oven to 350°F.

Combine flour, sugars, baking powder, baking soda, and sea salt into a small mixing bowl.

In a medium bowl mix together the bananas, peanut butter, Greek yogurt, egg, vanilla, and oil.

Fold in flour mixture until thoroughly combined and then gently fold in chocolate chips.

Pour the batter into a greased 9x5 inch loaf pan.

Bake for 30-45 minutes, or until toothpick comes out clean.

Cool in pan for 15 minutes. Carefully remove from pan and allow to cool completely on wire rack before slicing.

coconut macaroons

Makes about 25 small or 10-12 large macaroons

Preheat oven to 350°F.

Add egg whites and salt to a mixing bowl. Beat until egg whites form a stiff foam. Add powdered sugar a little bit at a time and mix well. Fold in coconut and vanilla extract.

Use an ice cream scoop to place a mound of mixture onto cookie sheets that have been lightly greased with virgin coconut oil. Bake for 15-20 minutes or until lightly browned. Remove from oven and let cool.

If making chocolate dipped macaroons, heat a double boiler* over medium high heat. Add dark chocolate chips to double boiler and stir until melted. Dip the bottom or sides of macaroon in chocolate and place on baking sheet lined with waxed paper.

Place in the refrigerator for 20 minutes or until chocolate hardens. May keep macaroons in refrigerator until ready to serve.

*A double boiler is a set of two fitted saucepans or pots that are stacked together with space between them. The bottom saucepan is filled with water, then the second saucepan is stacked on top. The steam from the bottom pot rises and heats the upper pot.

4 egg whites

Pinch of salt

¾ cup organic powdered sugar

8-ounce package unsweetened shredded coconut

1 teaspoon vanilla extract

1 tablespoon virgin coconut oil (to grease baking sheet)

2 ¾ cup organic white whole wheat flour

¼ teaspoon sea salt

1 teaspoon non-aluminum baking soda

1 ½ cups sugar*

1 stick organic grass-fed butter or ¾ cup virgin coconut oil

2 large organic free-range eggs

1 teaspoon organic 100% pure vanilla extract

Optional Cookie Add-Ins:

lemon juice and zest with lemon sugar**

oatmeal raisin***

organic sprinkles (made with vegetable/fruit-based food coloring)

kristen: My advice is to eat whatever you want as long as it's homemade. Have your cookies and eat them too!

so good sugar cookies

Makes about 20 cookies

Preheat oven to 350°F.

In a medium bowl stir together flour, salt, and baking soda. Set aside. In a large mixing bowl, cream together sugar and butter or oil. Blend in eggs, one at a time then add vanilla. Add flour mixture, one cup at a time, blending after each addition, until flour is incorporated.

If making different varieties, add preferred ingredients at this stage.

Refrigerate dough for one hour. Remove dough from refrigerator and use a cookie scoop to form dough into 2-inch balls. Place on non-greased cookie sheet. Using the bottom of a glass, press down lightly on each ball of dough until cookie is about ½ inch thick. (Use flour if dough starts to stick to bottom of glass). Bake cookies for 10-12 minutes and let cool before frosting.

*May substitute sugar with organic coconut sugar for a less sweet and darker color sugar cookie.

**Prepare lemon sugar by blending ½ cup sugar with 1 teaspoon lemon zest in a small food processor. Pulse until the lemon zest is incorporated into the sugar. After forming the dough balls as above, roll them in prepared lemon sugar Bake as instructed.

***Add 1/2 cup raisins and 1/2 cup oatmeal to cookie dough before refrigerating.

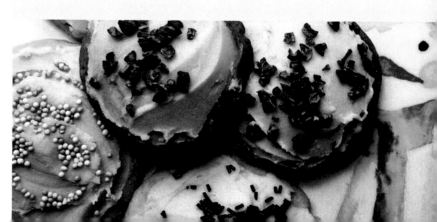

coconut butter frosting

Makes 2 cups of frosting

Combine virgin coconut oil, coconut manna, 1 cup of powdered sugar, and vanilla extract in a large bowl. Blend with a hand-held mixer until well combined.

While beater is running, add powdered sugar and milk alternately, ¼ cup at time until remainder of powdered sugar is used and frosting is desired consistency. Use more milk for a thinner frosting or icing consistency.

Use immediately or place frosting in refrigerator in an airtight container.

If using refrigerated frosting, let soften at room temperature for 1 hour before using. Frosting will last in the refrigerator for 4-5 days.

½ cup virgin coconut oil, softened

¼ cup coconut manna (coconut butter), softened

1 16-ounce package organic powdered sugar

1 tablespoon vanilla extract

½ to 1 cup original almond milk

tip ▶ Coconut Manna is made when dried coconut meat is ground into a very fine pulp resulting in a butter consistency. To use, warm the jar up in a pot of hot water and stir to combine. Coconut manna tends to have a richer flavor than virgin coconut oil and can be used in place of butter or nut butters.

whipped coconut cream

Serves 2

Place can of coconut milk in refrigerator for 2 hours so the cream separates from the coconut water.

Open the can and scoop out just the hardened cream that forms on the top and add to a mixing bowl. Save the remainder of the coconut water to use at another time.

Add vanilla extract to coconut cream and mix with a hand-held mixer until it achieves a whipped cream consistency.

1 can original coconut milk

1 teaspoon vanilla extract

tip ▶ The hardened cream that forms on the top of canned coconut milk makes for a delicious fluffy dessert topper.

banana ice cream

Serves 2

3 frozen bananas (peel and freeze overripe bananas for future use)

2 tablespoons cashew butter (can use any nut butter)

2 tablespoons dark cacao nibs

Cut frozen bananas into 1-inch slices.

Place in food processor and blend until creamy, about 30 seconds.

Add in cashew butter and blend to mix. Top with dark cacao nibs and enjoy!

Feel free to enjoy banana ice cream plain or add your own favorite toppings!

 Skip the ice cream and go for a banana ice cream instead! As the food processor blends the frozen bananas, it generates heat which causes the bananas to turn into a frozen yogurt consistency. Add your favorite toppings and enjoy a healthy sundae loaded with potassium, fiber, and antioxidants.

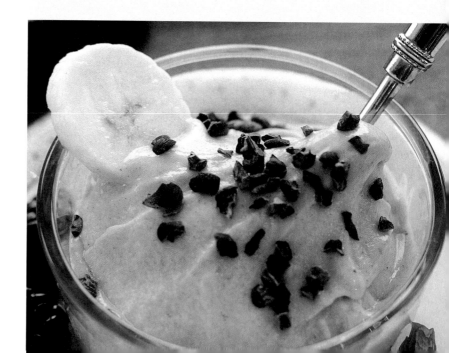

mandel bread (mandelbrot)

Makes 3 (8 inch) loaves

Preheat oven to 350°F.

Beat eggs, butter, sugar and vanilla in a large bowl. Add baking powder and flour, one cup at a time till mixed well. Add 1/2 cup of each of your desired add-ins and mix with a large spoon. Form mixture into a large dough ball, wrap with saran wrap and refrigerate overnight. To cook, remove from refrigerator and form dough into three, 8-inch loafs on a greased cooking sheet.

Bake for 35 minutes.

Let cool for 30 minutes before slicing into 1 inch pieces. Serve immediately or wrap in saran wrap and foil to freeze for later use.

4 eggs

1 stick organic unsalted butter, room temperature

1 cup organic sugar

2 teaspoons pure vanilla extract

2 teaspoons baking powder

3 cups organic unbleached all-purpose flour

Optional Add-Ins:

dark chocolate chips

cacao nibs

raisins

chopped nuts

dried cranberries

shredded coconut

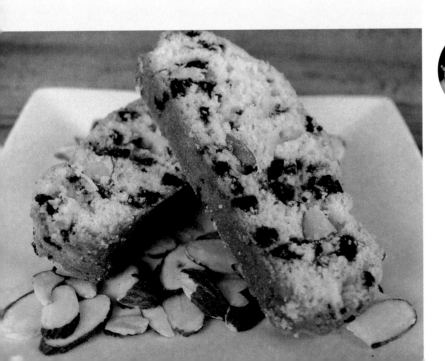

kristen: This delicious bready cookie, a recipe from my husband's Grandma Marilyn, is similar to biscotti and is a staple during family Hanukkah celebrations and many other special occasions. The Yiddish word, Mandelbrot means almond bread. Mondal is Yiddish for almond. Chocolate, nuts, and coconut make a delicious Mandel bread everyone is sure to love.

sherbet delight

Serves 4

10 ounces frozen strawberries

2 large bananas

4 dates (pitted)

½ cup raw almonds (soaked in water for 2 hours)

½ cup almond milk

Shredded coconut and cacao nibs for garnish

Combine all ingredients in a food processor and blend until smooth. Top with coconut and cacao nibs.

> Cacao nibs are a healthy magnesium-rich substitute for chocolate chips.

apple crisp

Serves 8

5 pounds apples, peeled and sliced

2 teaspoons cinnamon

2 cups rolled oats

1 cup whole wheat flour

¼ cup packed brown sugar

¼ teaspoon sea salt

1 teaspoon baking powder

2 eggs

½ cup organic virgin coconut oil, melted

Preheat oven to 325°F.

Toss apples with cinnamon and arrange in bottom of a 9x13 inch pan.

Mix dry ingredients together in a medium bowl.

Lightly beat eggs and add to dry ingredients. Gently work in eggs until mixture is crumbly.

Spread mixture on top of apples.

Pour melted virgin coconut oil evenly over the top of the mixture.

Bake 1 hour.

> Cinnamon is considered a super spice and is especially beneficial for balancing blood sugar and keeping energy level steady.

raw banana pecan pie

Serves 8

To make the crust:

Grind the first 3 ingredients in a food processor until finely ground. Press mixture evenly into an 8-inch pie dish.

To make the filling:

Blend dates, overripe bananas, and lemon juice in the food processor until smooth.

Fold in banana slices and pour combined mixture into the pie crust.

Sprinkle about 1 tablespoon of chopped pecans on top, cover with plastic wrap, and refrigerate for a couple hours.

For the crust:

1 cup raw pecans

1 cup dates, pitted

½ teaspoon vanilla extract

For the filling:

5 dates, pitted

3 overripe bananas

1 tablespoon fresh lemon juice

1 banana, sliced

1 tablespoon pecans, chopped

tip ▶ To make raw pie crusts, simply use a 1:1 ratio of dried fruit to nuts.

spirulina birthday pie

Serves 8

For the crust:

2 cups raw almonds, finely ground in food processor

⅓ cup dried figs, chopped (2-3 figs)

1 tablespoon agave nectar or raw honey

For the filling:

¾ cup coconut water

¼ cup raw cashews

¼ cup virgin coconut oil

1 tablespoon agave nectar or raw honey

1 tablespoon crushed spirulina and chlorella tablets

Toppings:

1 tablespoon cacao nibs

Nuts of choice

To make the crust:

Combine ground almonds and figs in a food processor and pulse until fine crumbles.

Transfer almond fig mixture to a mixing bowl.

Add agave nectar and mix well to form a crust like consistency. Press the crust mixture evenly into the bottom and sides of an 8-inch pie tin.

For the filling:

Combine all of the filling ingredients in a high-speed blender or food processor and blend until smooth.

Pour the mixture into the pie crust and top with cacao nibs and your favorite nuts.

Freeze for at least one hour or overnight.

Remove from freezer 20 minutes before serving.

kristen: *No one should go without spirulina pie on their birthday! I make this for my dad every year. It is a true superfood dessert.*

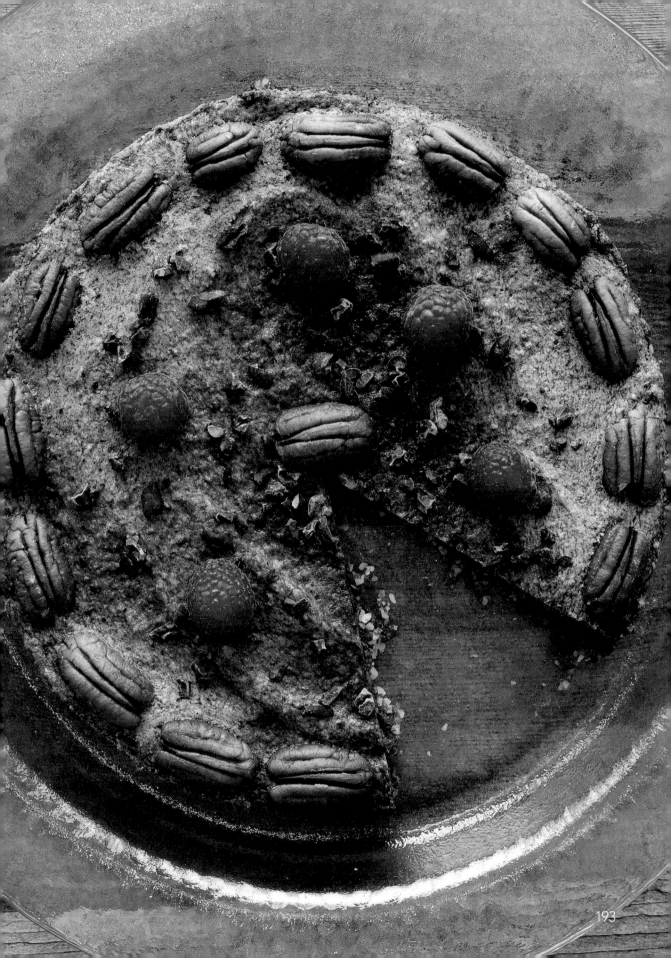

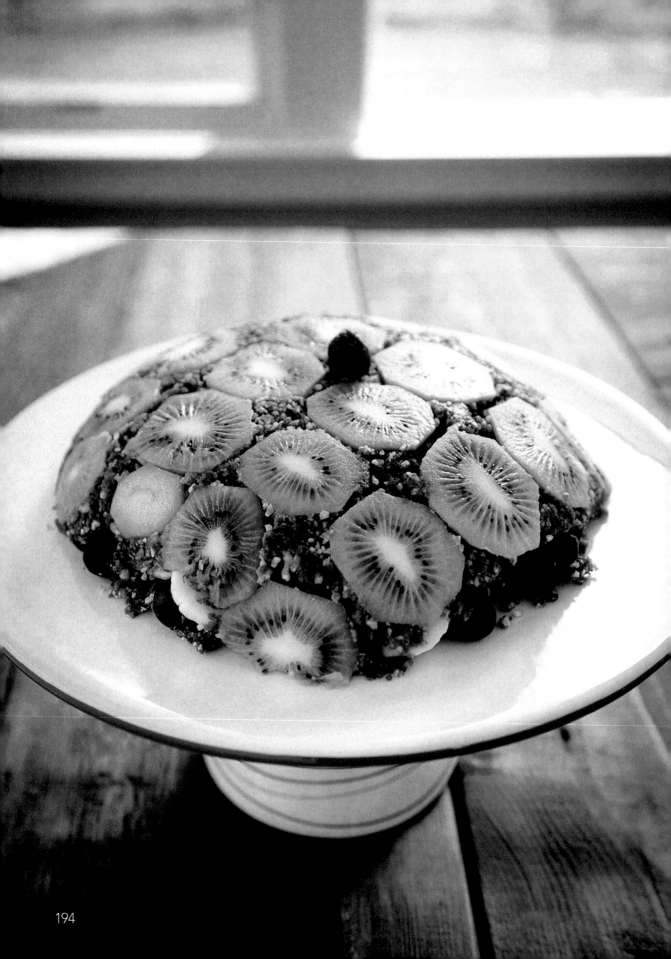

fruity delicious upside down cake

Serves 4

Combine the pecans, dates, and vanilla in a food processor and pulse until finely ground.

Line a small mixing bowl with saran wrap. The bowl should be approximately 7 inches wide, by 3½ inches deep to allow ingredient layers to be seen when served.

Layer kiwi slices in rows along bottom and up the sides of bowl.

Press half of the pecan and date mixture evenly over the kiwi slices to secure in place. Push date mixture in the spaces between the kiwi slices.

Layer banana slices, blueberries and raspberries over the pressed pecans and dates.

Cover the fruit layers with the second half of the pecan and date mixture, and press to seal.

Push down so the top is level with the edges.

Wrap in saran wrap and place in refrigerator for 20 minutes to set.

To serve, remove top layer of saran and place serving dish on bowl. Flip the bowl and plate, and remove the bowl from the filling. Remove saran wrap.

Cut into slices and serve.

 Nothing is sweeter than nature's candy. Perfectly wrapped and oh so delicious!

2 cups raw pecans

2 cups pitted dates

1 teaspoon vanilla extract

2-3 kiwis, peeled and sliced

1-2 bananas, sliced

1 pint blueberries

1 pint raspberries

 kristen: For a special touch, buy organic whipping cream and whip it yourself with a little vanilla extract for a delicious cake topper!

index

f

g

y

z

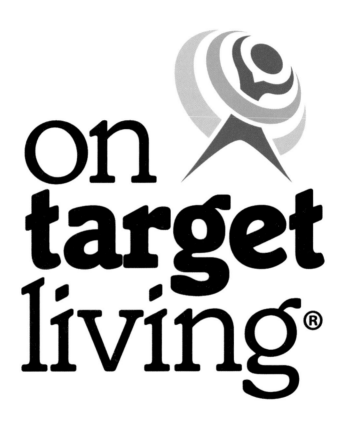

ontargetliving.com   #targettotable

GETTING HEALTHIER STARTS WITH COOKING MORE MEALS AT HOME

Cooking stimulates all 5 of our senses to make us feel complete and satisfied. It's said that the more we tap into our senses, the greater potential we have for enjoying life.

At On Target Living we teach a lifestyle that is not only centered around foods that nourish the body and improve health but that also incorporates daily movement and proper rest and rejuvenation to build your whole self. REST, EAT, and MOVE are the foundation of On Target Living and helping you discover the power of feeling your best.

On Target Living is a lifestyle designed to help people reach optimal health, balance, energy and vitality through:

- Prioritizing rest and rejuvenation
- Developing healthy eating habits
- Incorporating exercise into daily routines

On Target Living provides the resources and knowledge to improve:

- Cholesterol balance
- Weight loss
- Type 2 Diabetes
- Blood Pressure
- Acid Reflux
- Digestion
- Hormonal health
- Sleep
- Energy
- Auto-immune issues
- Allergies

On Target Living works with leading organizations around the world to expand human capacity and improve health and performance through:

- Keynotes / Presentations
- Trainings
- Retreats
- Coaching
- Products
- Educational Resources

Find these products and more at: shop.ontargetliving.com

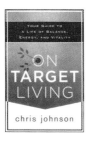
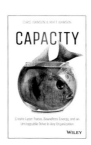
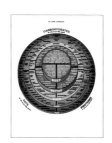
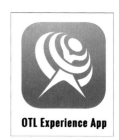

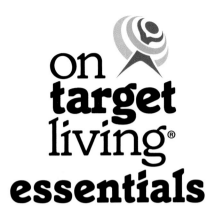

on target living® essentials

OFFERING THE BEST
SO YOU CAN FEEL YOUR BEST

On Target Living Essentials are products we believe are "essential" for optimal health, performance and well-being. We source only the best quality products on the market, conveniently gathered in one location and delivered right to your door.

At shop.ontargetliving.com you will find:

- Nutrient dense superfoods including wheatgrass, spirulina/chlorella, cod liver oil, virgin coconut oil, hemp seeds, flax seeds, chia seeds, cacao nibs, and so much more.

- Educational resources designed to teach, inspire, and motivate you to live your best.

To learn more about On Target Living's services, products, and free resources, visit **ontargetliving.com**